i-MINDS

How Cell Phones, Computers, Gaming, and Social Media Are Changing Our Brains, Our Behavior, and the Evolution of Our Species

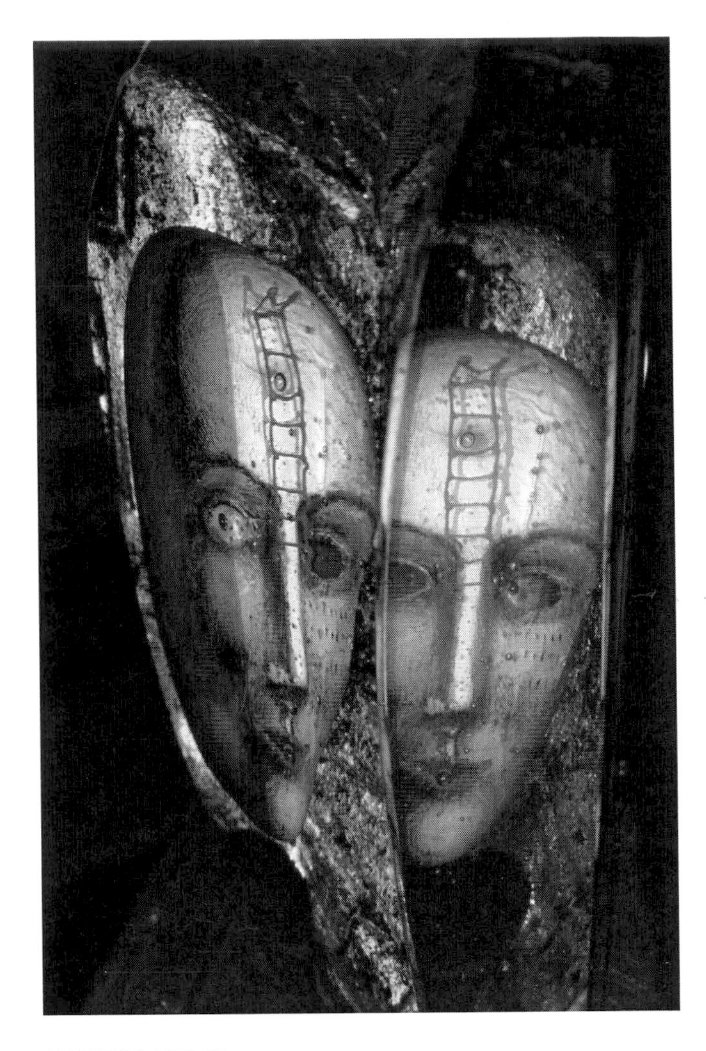

JANUS'S LADDER
by Bertil Vallien, Swedish sculptor and glass artist.

www.bertilvallien.se, www.vidamuseum.com

Reproduction permission generously granted by the artist.
Photograph by Christian Cederroth

Janus in Roman Mythology is the God of beginnings and transition. Janus has two faces as he looks equally to the future as to the past.

i-Minds

How Cell Phones, Computers, Gaming, and Social Media Are Changing Our Brains, Our Behavior, and the Evolution of Our Species

MARI K. SWINGLE, PhD

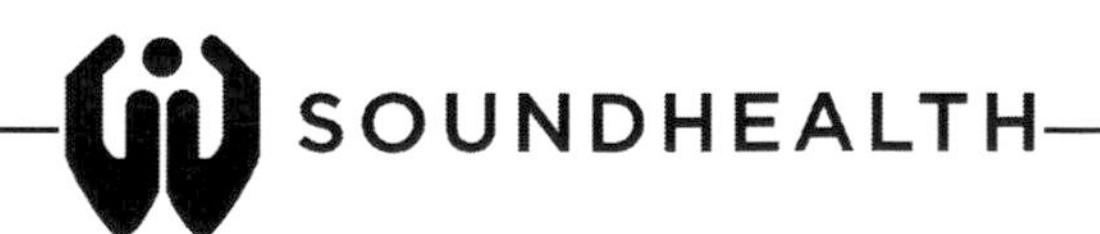

Cover and interior design by Masha Shubin
Janus's Ladder by Bertil Vallien, photo by Christian Cederroth
Author photo by Christian Cederroth
Cover Images (BigStockPhoto.com): Apple Profile Bites © Metsafile; Shining Green Yellow Printed Circuit Board © MastakA.

Publisher: Inkwater Press | www.inkwaterpress.com

ISBN 978-0-9810800-1-7

Printed in Canada.

3 5 7 9 10 8 6 4 2

Table of Contents

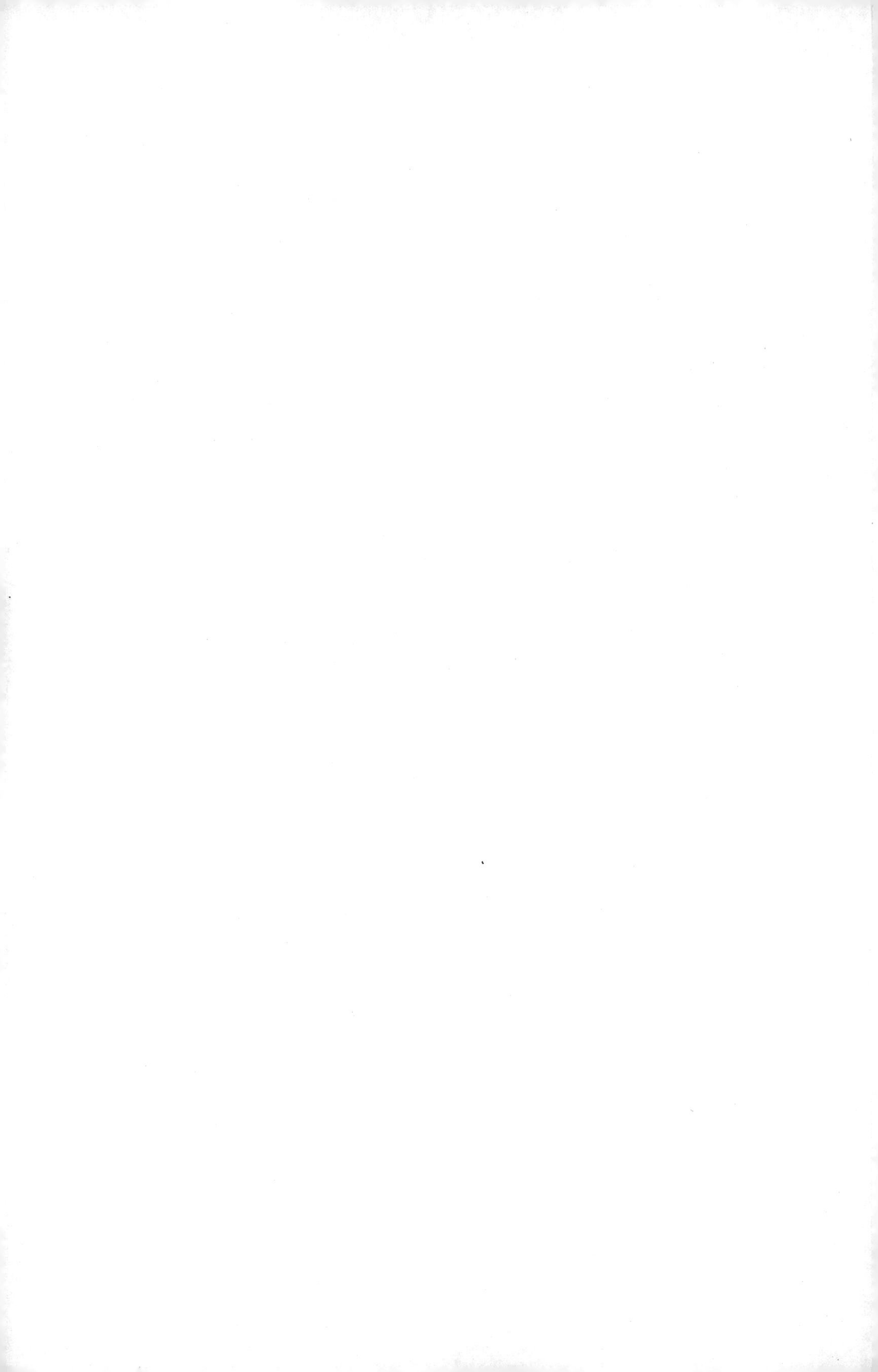

Introduction

Societal Shifting

Every era has an innovation that changes the face of society: the way we think, the way we act and interact as individuals, as a community, and as a culture. As the innovation is introduced, it tends to be greeted with elation. As the innovation becomes integrated and the first societal shifts become apparent, some start to question the balance of benefit and loss in the equation of change. We are now in such a place with digital media.

Cellphones, PCs, and the Internet are now completely integrated in global culture, i-culture: welcomed by most, resisted by some, the impact apparent for all. There is great change for the better, but now, a few decades into the assimilation, there is also arguably evidence of an equally negative impact. The darker side of the digital era has emerged.

Be it due to naiveté or denial, the negative influences of digital media are expanding, blindly accepted by most – educators, business, parents, and partners, who later wonder what went terribly wrong. This book will explore such changes and hopefully provide food for thought on what we should embrace and accept, what we should unequivocally reject, and the many aspects of the digital era that we should now be debating.

The debate, unfortunately, often gets sidetracked into generational arguments – a generational divide wherein the older complain of the younger becoming progressively stupid, rude, and isolating with i-tech at the expense of interpersonal or face-to-face relationships. The young, like any generation before, equally find their pre–i-tech elders ignorant of advancement, judgmental, invasive, and abrasive in their views, feeling they should stop pontificating and get with the times. But we are all missing the point. By sticking staunchly to our positions we risk missing the fine print: the subtle and not so subtle changes in human behavior and underlying brain function that are unequivocally changing all that we are, and the world that we live in. Here we all owe it to ourselves, and the generations that will follow, to open our eyes, look up, and examine change in action, to arm ourselves with information on who we are, and what we wish to become in this new, and yes, wonderful, i-mediated world.

...and now the dark side

First Hints of a Problem

Over the past two decades, a select group of scholars and health care practitioners began to systematically note the emergence of a new set of issues seemingly associated with excessive usage and otherwise unhealthy applications of i-technologies. Today the effects are confirmed, notably in the realms of sexuality, socialization, education, and failure to launch. For children, adolescents, and youth, excessive usage of digital media is now highly associated with learning disabilities, emotional dysregulation, as well as conduct or behavioral disorders. For adults, it is highly correlated with anxiety, depression, sexual dysfunction and sexual deviation, insomnia, social isolation, disaffected pair bonding, marital conflict, and compromised work performance. In clinical practice I am also starting to note some rather frightening connections with thwarted emotional and cognitive development in the very young.

Opening Our Eyes

I would like to think we are wiser now as a global culture, having learned from past mistakes, that we no longer blindly continue on paths of innovation without looking up to examine the potential toll. My last eighteen years working in a clinical environment, however, are telling me otherwise. Unlike excessive consumption or abuse of other substances such as alcohol, food, or drugs, for many, the effects of excessive usage of digital media are rarely perceived as contributing to, never mind as causing a specific ailment, condition, or conflict.

All this said, digital media is here to stay and has unquestionably advanced our world. It is not negative by nature. This is not the claim that this book will make; not by far. But what the Internet and all digital media give, they can also take away. How we use it, interact with it, and depend on it vis-à-vis our "real" world and real relationships within are key.

The questions we now need to start asking ourselves are not what the technologies are positively contributing, as these contributions are rather evident, but rather what the technologies are replacing or taking away: an older technology, a behavior, a skill, a relationship, our compassion, values...intelligence? It is time to widen our focus to the broader effects of i-technology in all the branches of our day-to-day lives. It is time to ask ourselves what i-media is truly facilitating.

In This Book

This book is written from a clinician's perspective. As a practicing psychologist, and a certified neurotherapist, I have based *i-Minds* upon what has crossed my clinical floor: how i-media is affecting children, partners, family, learning. The list is long.

Weaving through larger societal shifts, including history, research and hard data, developmental theory, literature on brain function and mental illness, professional reflections, popular literature, and observations from clinical practice, I will illustrate how the medium is influencing our thinking and our processing – our functioning as a whole.

I will look at micro-cultures, such as high school and bullying, parenting circles, and dating, as well as shifts in macro-culture affecting work, sexuality, mental health, learning, play, creative process, attachment, and development itself. I will explore the increase in apathy and general hyper-arousal in the masses associated with excessive applications of i-tech. I will also explore the extreme: a new and growing phenomenon threatening to become the addiction of the twenty-first century, referred to as Internet Addiction (IA), Digital Addiction, or i-addiction.

The i-phenomenon will be explored in tandem from three distinct angles.

- First, I will explore the big picture of what is affecting us all, regardless of age, gender, culture, or creed.

- I will also present what appears to be generation specific – not exclusively by chronological age itself, but rather by age as it relates to the rate of the assimilation of the technologies.

- Lastly, I will discuss the effects of digital media in terms of level of immersion: the way, or more specifically the "why" and the "how" some of us are using the medium to the inclusion or exclusion of other activities or relationships.

For those of you who are more scientifically or research oriented, supplemental details are presented in sections labeled ***Scientific Corner***. For those of you who are not, these sections can be skipped without losing the general flow. Definitions of some potentially unfamiliar terms and key points will also be included within the text in italics.

Interspersed throughout, I will sprinkle advice: solutions, options, and actions one can choose to follow if situations and vignettes seem all too familiar. My goal is to educate, to ensure that i-tech remains a solid complement to all that we are, integrated with but not overriding the human element in cognition and development, work, industry, education, socialization, and play.

Great Beginnings

Subtle Shifts in Behavior

But first, how did this all start?

The World Wide Web, as we first called it, was a military innovation that, when it crossed over into civilian life, was embraced as changing the world only for the better. Indeed, in its beginnings, it was most positive. First gaining a foothold in academic communities in the early 1990s, the Internet was the ideal tool for research and learning.[1] Soon, no more restrictions on library hours, no more trudging across campus only to find someone else had reserved the book or article you needed. It was also the ideal form of international communication. No more fallen land lines, outrageous telephone bills, and one could see, never mind merely talk to, colleagues, friends, and family while traveling or studying away from home.

The Web, as promptly nicknamed, was a most novel and efficient form of communication; it was not location-specific, and was accessible for free with any PC and phone line. In the 1990s many of us had, and used, university-funded email and later messaging, as the most efficient form of communication long before we had, or could afford, cell phones.

It soon became apparent, however, that the Internet was also changing "local" behavior. In my own graduate school experience, friends started sending diatribes of thought via email. Discussions we would usually have gathered for and debated over a coffee or a beer were now sequential monologues sent via computer. Although initially most entertaining, some of us, including myself, noted the reduction of face-to-face social interaction and felt something was amiss. Although I did not precisely see it for what it was at the time, I was remotely aware of the development of a bit of a void. I, for one, was missing the reward or pleasure of the face-to-face social engagement.

Thereafter, some of us became quite engrossed in these great email dialogues, others less – still choosing to gather weekly in person. A small, and at the time barely notable division of social behaviors, and hence social circles, started within our tiny university network.

Viewed in retrospect, my experience as a master's student in the mid-1990s was not unique. Very early on, anecdotal reports started to emerge that indeed the Internet was changing social behavior. A rather amusing incident in circulation was how a group of international students was observed in a dorm, laughing and engaging, each with their own PC, rather than socializing with each other. At the time, we found this behavior peculiar and, hence, the story amusing. Why would you choose to play with a computer or communicate with others abroad, when you had friends, company, sitting right next to you? The end of the story was, for its time, a seemingly perfect double twist. Indeed these students were socializing with each other. They were not engaging at all with friends from abroad, but rather with each other in the same room via computer interface.

At the time, the behavior raised some eyebrows, but was also simply attributed to the harmless pursuit of novelty of the new medium. What we did not see, however, was that this was a great foreshadowing of things to come, something none of us, at the time, would ever have dreamed of. Now, merely twenty years later, this behavior is not unusual at all: digital interface has become the primary mode of communication for all youth.

From Subtle to Extreme – First Hints of Problematic Usage

Beyond amusement, very early on, it was noted that high Internet usage could also have quite serious detrimental effects.[2] Parallel to my own graduate school observation of social division, for some, Internet usage was leading to social avoidance and isolation as opposed to broader socialization networks, albeit done under the precise illusion of communication and social interaction.

Similarly, in academia, the ideal tool for research and scholarship was negatively affecting academic performance and class attendance. Students were skipping class and handing in assignments late, having stayed up too late playing or "researching" on the Web. For a select group, time that was previously dedicated to work, school, chores, or social interaction with family, friends, and peers was now dedicated to Internet usage – to the neglect of other activities and interactions.

The medium was showing potential to have exactly the opposite of its intended effect: reducing, as opposed to broadening, the scope of socialization, work, scholastic, and general life efficiency. For some academics, questions started to arise as to whether this form of excessive Internet usage had the properties of addiction.[3,4,5,6,7] The answer now, over twenty years later, is clearly "yes."

As with all forms of addiction, some forms of excess are decidedly black and white. But what about the proverbial shades of gray? How, and when, do we mark a behavior crossing from positive to negative, from neutral to destructive? In contrast, when should we adapt? When is change itself a mere sign of change of the times?

Raising Our Awareness of Impact

A good way to examine present influence is to take lessons from the past. Picture the arrival, or more importantly, the assimilation, of any of the great innovations of the last century (e.g., the telephone, television, car, or the airplane). They all have brought great benefit and some questionable shifts. The car is an ideal example;

the advantages need not be mentioned as they are vast. The negatives, such as the ecological footprint and contribution to lack of fitness and obesity, are equally known. But what of the more subtle and compounding influences that contribute to the positive and negative shift of an entire culture as a whole? For example, few of us consider the car's central influence on massive amendments in our management of time and our expectations of travel distance.

An apt illustration of the car's central role in mass societal change is the development of suburbia. In the mid-twentieth century, the automobile was promoted as the means to an affordable family home for all, a pleasant drive away from the bustling city. This new personal form of transportation was the turnkey to the North American dream: poetic images of quiet neighborhoods, children playing in the streets, fresh laundry flapping in the clean air in massive backyards.

Within less than thirty years, however, this dream for many slowly shifted into a nightmare. It slowly metamorphosed into a daily 1.5-hour, two-way commute – three hours per day, fifteen hours every week – time sacrificed to the method, the transportation that initially made it, the dream, possible.

This theft of time is now accepted by many of us as standard. We accept the method that now takes us away from family, from friends: leaving us with less personal, or leisure, time. The driving of greater and greater distances to take children to school, to soccer practice, to "play dates," is customary. Part of the reason kids don't play spontaneously in groups anymore is peer groups simply live too far apart.

The wheels spin further: the loss of hours per day to transportation has led to the perceived need to purchase and consume fast food, frozen dinners, and canned soups (all sorts of pre-prepared and processed foods) as no one any longer has the time, or energy, to cook, let alone share a meal together. The perceived need now for two cars per nuclear family has resulted in accumulated debt, financial strain, and more work hours needed to pay for it all. We are far, far away from a cruise into work and a leisurely Sunday afternoon drive.

Plugging In

Similarly, the digital era crept into our lives. The PC, then laptop, email, and the personal cell phone were all welcomed as godsends: tools that would change the global workplace in terms of logistic limitations and communicative efficiency. They would liberate us from our desks and eliminate distance with virtual time.

All this did happen, but what also happened, identical to the automobile, is that digital media's blessing also became its curse. The universal place-time accessibility we initially embraced thereafter systematically invaded all aspects of our lives. We are now always "on call": workers, parents, spouses, children, lovers, all of us in (all) our multiple roles. Many of us now do not, or cannot, liberate ourselves from "accessibility" and the buzz of the world.

But what is this doing to our brains?

The short answer is that our brains are speeding up, but not in a good way. Our neurophysiological reaction, or functional adaptation, to the age of digital media is a higher state of arousal and the nemesis that comes with. What nemesis? Quite simply, higher states of arousal come with decreased abilities to self-quiet. Elevated states of arousal are further coupled with a reduced ability to self-stimulate and self-entertain. This includes reduced abilities to observe, integrate information, and to be creative. In essence, we have less ability to sustain focus on the normal, the baseline, including states of observation, contemplation, and transitions from which ideas spark – what many under the age of twenty now consider a void, proclaiming boredom.

The short answer is that our brains are speeding up, but not in a good way. Our neurophysiological reaction, or functional adaptation, to the age of digital media is a higher state of arousal.

We now feel agitated when not externally stimulated; we need to be occupied, entertained. We also have greater troubles quieting, including reaching states of repose, satisfaction, and restorative sleep.

The implications of this are vast. On a biological as well as a cultural level, such brain state changes affect learning, socialization, recreation, partnering, parenting, and creativity – in essence all factors that make a society and a culture. The neurophysiological processes that regulate mood and behavior are deregulating. What we are left with is massive behavioral-biological, and hence, cultural, shifting. Placing this in the map of disorders or pathology we now see that excessive usage of digital media has a concrete relationship to ADHD, Autism, and mood deregulation including anxiety, depression, and anger management, other forms of addiction, and all behaviors on the obsessive-compulsive spectrum.

i-MINDS

How Cell Phones, Computers, Gaming, and Social Media Are Changing Our Brains, Our Behavior, and the Evolution of Our Species

CHAPTER ONE

Technological Integration Versus Technological Interference

How Do We Know If We Have a Budding Problem?

For many of us i-tech is a wonderful tool facilitating all that life has to offer. For others i-tech negatively affects work, relationships, and mental health, generally thwarting our well-being as well as that of those close to us. The way digital technologies affect us can vary immensely, as can the reasons why. Stripped down, everything is of influence: our age, gender, ethnicity, sexual orientation and identification, occupation, family dynamics, personality, state of mental health and happiness...It is potentially an endless list.

All that said, determining if our usage is healthy or unhealthy boils down to two simple questions: First, to what extent are we immersed in digital technologies and why? Second, is our usage integrated or interfering? Problems stem from why and how we use the medium, not if we do or don't use it.

As will be reviewed later, modalities and measurement systems now exist that can assist in determining if the use of digital media has a potential to be problematic. For many of us, however, warning signs emerge long, long, before a problem is defined. On the slippery slope from unhealthy usage to full blown i-addiction, hints of depression (e.g., negativity, apathy, and withdrawing) or anxiety (edginess, sleeplessness, and moodiness) are signs of which one should be leery. True to most budding addictions though, the cascading pre-addict is frequently in a heavy state of denial. Untrue of other addictions, however, in Internet or Digital Addiction, family, employees, and community tend be significantly less aware. Many of us are also personally or culturally further unwittingly enabling the problematic usage.

What i-Problem?

There tend to be two presentations of problematic usage profiles. In the first, an individual's excessive use is overt but not identified as central or contributing to a problem (*referred to as denial and naïve presentation*) and, of course, there is covert (*hidden*) use.

That said, very rarely is usage itself overtly identified as "the" problem itself. Case in point, at the clinic where I practice, excessive use of i-tech tends not to be reported at intake for either children or adults. Individuals present for another concern such as poor scholastic performance, suspicion of ADHD, anxiety, depression, conduct disorder, insomnia, concerns regarding bullying or social isolation, marital conflict, etc. Excessive i-usage is not even on the radar.

Until recently these clients were a bit of an enigma. They did not respond to therapy as did others. Some would report no changes or very slight changes despite weeks of intervention. Others would report dramatic changes and subsequently regress completely. And then, there was inevitably an epiphany wherein it became apparent that excessive use of digital media had a compounding, if not central, role in symptoms. Excessive usage was key in the development or maintenance of the primary ailment or issue for which the individual or their family initially sought psychological services. But why did no one see this?

One explanation is that unlike many other problematic behaviors or addictions, inappropriate or unhealthy usage of digital media can easily fly under the radar. As was noted, at the very beginning of the phenomenon, excessive and unhealthy applications can be easily masked by legitimate work or scholastic pursuits (e.g., research) as well as otherwise harmless social behavior (e.g., Facebooking, texting, and tweeting). In the case of adults, another sociological factor contributing to the spread of the phenomenon is the value much of modern society places on sacrifice for work, or career martyrdom.

A Tale of Two Men

Take for example two men sharing stories at the office coffee machine. The first man, let's call him Jeff, laments how he stayed extremely late in an attempt to finish an important project. Only when absolutely exhausted did he head home. Having no time to spare to eat, he grabbed a burger at a drive-through. Once home, he said a quick "hello" to his wife and daughter before secluding himself in the den and resuming the project. Finally, project still unfinished, he took himself exhausted to bed at 3 a.m. The following day he laments (and boasts) to his office colleagues how it is only dedication that got him up on time to get to work. He hopes he can finish by the deadline at noon.

The second man, let's say Steve, shares how he felt he did a good enough job yesterday and was quite comfortable leaving the project at 5 p.m. Now, he is fit to resume. Being well-rested and in a good mood, Steve believes with a few uninterrupted hours he will surely finish by mid-morning. Steve tells of how he had a mostly pleasant evening at home with his family, cooking and sharing a lovely meal. He had a bit of a homework struggle with his daughter that blew out of proportion, but hey, that's kids and to be expected from time to time. He then took some personal time on the computer, searching the entertainment listings, stocks, and daily news, then went to bed, including lovemaking with his wife (a detail perhaps not shared with colleagues).

Ask yourself which man will get the social reward (empathy, support, or praise) for "dedication" to his work. Also, ask yourself which man was most likely distracting himself from his work, or entertaining himself otherwise, online at work as well as at home. Chances are that Jeff was systematically entertaining himself, or distracting himself, with other online activities under the guise of work at his computer. This secondary use, not the complexity of project itself, was the cause of being behind on the project – and everyone (including him), "fell for it."

Turning Bad

The best way to establish if an individual has a problem is to determine whether usage is negatively interfering with work, school, or relationships. In the above example, Steve's usage would be clearly integrated: positive or neutral. His use of digital technologies did not interfere with his two primary relationships (his daughter and wife), nor did it interfere with his work. He was available for family cohesiveness as well as chores (family dinner and clean-up), parental duty (homework and behavioral struggle with daughter), and romance/intimacy within his partnership. He was also on schedule with his project at work. He used technology for personal time as well as perhaps for future social time (searching entertainment listings).

Jeff, on the other hand, was behind schedule at work, sacrificed his two primary relationships, including his parental duty, as well as his own health (fast food). It is highly likely that there will be consequences in his primary relationships (e.g., his wife becoming resentful of his absence and her double parental duty, and his daughter feeling abandoned and/or alienated from her father). Jeff's "work" was undoubtedly a cover for a multitude of other online activities. If his pattern is systematically repeated, there will be consequences at his work as well as compromised family dynamics, including marital strife and greater potential for future behavioral issues with his daughter.

Change of the Times

The tale of these two men is a clear example of technological integration versus technological interference. It is also an example common to what can be referred to as the first generation of digital users.

There are a few generations of the digital age. As will be discussed in chapters following, there are also accordingly different phases of amalgamation and accompanying neurophysiological adaptation. For now, however, I will speak of what Prensky[8] and others refer to as Digital Immigrants versus Digital Natives. Digital immigrants are my generation and older (late forties BTW). We are termed "immigrants" as we were not born into digital culture: we moved into it. My generation grew up with TV and land lines (AKA telephones attached to walls). If you were lucky as a teenager, you might have had a jack in your bedroom allowing for some privacy in conversation; otherwise you spoke to all, under the eyes of all, in the kitchen or living room. Until we were well into our mid-twenties, PCs and cell phones were from the land of the supremely wealthy or our childhood science fiction (e.g., *Star Trek* and *Dr. Who*).

Perhaps of equal importance in my generation is how each of us chose to assimilate. True to how immigrants behave, some of us leapt into the new era while others stood in trepidation on the sidelines, observing. Some of us even staunchly stood to preserve our way of life, our culture of origin, leaving the cultural change to occur in the second, or native, generation. But one advantage digital immigrants do have is that of perspective: we all have been witness to great changes in ourselves and the generation(s) that came after us. Most of us note surface changes, for example, what we perceive of as a shallowness of information, a subtle lack of depth and length of conversation, of attention: staccato of sorts, as opposed to a melody in personal interaction.

More in depth, I feel extremely blessed to have been working in a branch of applied psychology (*electroencephalography and neurotherapy, a branch of psychology involving brain mapping and its treatment modality*) during this time of great transition. Working primarily with children and families, I have been able to observe first hand not only the changes in behaviors but the changes in neurophysiology and the associated psychological complaints associated with the assimilation of i-tech. From this vantage point, I can confidently speak of three generations or phases of neurological and associated behavioral change.[9] These changes clearly relate to the broadness of integration and the depth of immersion of the individual in the macro and micro culture of the technologies.

The story of Jeff and Steve tends to be one of digital immigrants, where one individual has clearly fallen prey to the medium while the other has not. Steve's usage is healthy, and integrated, while Jeff's is at best avoidant and interfering. Now, in the third decade of amalgamation, we also have some understanding of "why."

Psychosocial Instability and Poor Assimilation of Digital Immigrants

From a psychosocial perspective, it is highly likely that Steve was a well-adjusted and otherwise content individual, hence naturally merging or integrating the new technologies into his work and personal life and taking advantage of the advancement and the convenience of the medium. Jeff, on the other hand, was most likely experiencing some sort of psychological or social difficulty, for example, a mild depression or budding anxiety, perhaps an intimacy issue, or another sub-clinical pathology (*a mental disorder that is not quite strong enough yet to seek medical or psychiatric attention*). These sub-clinical problems are central factors in the development of problematic applications of the technologies,[10] as is what an individual chooses to do next.

> In the case of problematic usage of i-technologies, instead of seeking professional help, or otherwise communicating mental, physical, or emotional unrest to family or friends, individuals seek some sort of solace, or shelter, in escaping to i-media.

The second factor that ensures the

development of a problem is to whom, or rather to "what," the individual turns to next. In the case of problematic usage of i-technologies, instead of seeking professional help, or otherwise communicating mental, physical, or emotional unrest to family or friends, individuals seek some sort of solace, or shelter, in escaping to i-media. And here is where a problem not only blossoms, but starts to grow roots. In what we now know is the catch of the medium, different from many other distracting activities or avoidance strategies, escaping to i-tech will exacerbate, rather than solve (or soothe) an individual's original problem.

Observations of the Digital Immigrants

Observing what can happen within our own generation(s) is one thing. Observing that which comes with the next can be quite another...

Digital Natives – How Can We Tell Normal Change from What Is Problematic?

Anyone over thirty who has ridden public transportation lately (or heck, even looked at their kids in the back seat of their car) will notice what, to them, is a new behavior. Just as foreshadowed by the story of the international students in the Introduction, some teens and youth don't appear to talk directly to, or with, each other anymore. Communication appears completely mediated by technology. Youth share ear buds, send each other messages, Snapchat, laugh over and share content looked up, sent, and received. But they rarely converse directly without some form of i-device.

Is this due to novelty? Is it just plain fun? Does it serve an explicit purpose such as keeping those not in the group on a bus or subway line in the social loop? Or do kids, like any generation before, just do things a little differently than their parents? The larger question or concern of course is whether this is the beginning of an innocuous sociological shift or are these the first explicit signs of a generation no longer capable of communicating with each other without a digital mediator?

Prensky, and others, speak of preferred methods of socialization (and learning) in digital natives. I would like to potentially challenge the semantics of this: asking how we differentiate a preference from an emergent dependence? Is this "new" behavior a sign of integration and expansion of communication style, or is the use of technological interface interfering with the learning of social bridging in an otherwise typically rather awkward stage of adolescence? In sum, is technology interfering with healthy social development in youth?

Defining Problematic

Before we further explore what makes consumption of digital media problematic, it might first be helpful to define non-problematic. Non-problematic usage is true integration. The technology fits in, being integral to modern life, without overriding, or eclipsing, the development, or maintenance, of other healthy behaviors, or relationships. Back to the story of Steve and Jeff; if Steve pulled out an iPhone at dinner to confirm an unfamiliar term his daughter learned in science class, it would be appropriate. He is using digital technology as a tool to facilitate comprehension or communication. In contrast, if Jeff interrupted his daughter, not letting her try to explain the term, choosing instead to look it up on his own, it would not. In doing this second action, Jeff would override his daughter's voice, and their relationship, for the instrument, and the technology – again integration versus interference. Interference has many other subtle compounding effects. Jeff's choice of action, for example, also risks compromising both the father-daughter relationship and his daughter's learning. It further compromises the development of patience and attentiveness in the listening–being heard dynamic between father and daughter, as well as his daughter's learning to communicate efficaciously in new or unfamiliar (knowledge) territory, in this case, in language or terminology newly learned in science class.

Integration, or progress, is when a technology, due to superior efficiency, replaces other methods, or expands a desired trait. Interference is when a technology overrides a desirable trait or eclipses a developmental phase.

Back to one of i-tech's primary applications, communication: using i-tech devices while on the move, or over distances, can be a most positive application that keeps us connected and has the bonus of facilitating daily life. In the case of the above example of adolescents on public transport, if interacting through digital media is one method or communication tool of many, it is entirely innocuous, and those of us resisting had indeed better get with the times. However, if it replaces or eliminates eye-to-eye communication, or overrides the development of states and traits including observation, patience, and developing the ability to be comfortable in silence, we should be cautious.

Integration, or progress, is when a technology, due to superior efficiency, replaces other methods, or expands a desired trait. Interference is when a technology overrides a desirable trait or eclipses a developmental phase.

Lastly, if youth can't do without, meaning they can't communicate, become nervous or agitated, in addition to bored, without their digital devices, this is a warning of developmental, if not pathological, change.

Cautions

When we are critiquing the dimensions of digital media and their influence on human behavior, it is key that a new technology not be blamed for, or confused with, personality traits, couple or family dynamics, or developmental stages that would exist, regardless. For a couple with communication problems, for example, the reading of, or rather the hiding behind, a newspaper over breakfast in the

1950s, or the television in the 1970s, would be equally problematic to Internet or i-tech usage today. The wall is present irrespective of the technology. Equally, a teenager does not need an iPhone, YouTube, or a gaming device to ignore or disrespect a parent. Parents are graced with this developmental stage regardless of digital media.

Three Types of Transformation and When to Start Questioning

Apart from the larger concerns of technologies interfering with natural phases of social or psychological development, we should be wary of three forms of psychosocial transformation.

1. In my clinical experience, the first form of problematic, or negative, application of digital media involves the medium *facilitating accentuation, or acceleration of a negative, or previously neutral, behavior*. An example of acceleration of the negative in adolescence would be when a small high school clique's bullying becomes a massive attack of cyberbullying crossing social groups, schools, and even neighborhoods. An example of transformation of a relatively neutral to a negative behavior is when normal teenage sexual curiosity (e.g., watching some porn online) evolves into sexual deviance (e.g., becoming a voyeur). In both cases, the behaviors (bullying and sexual curiosity) already exist, but digital media functions as the tool of negative magnification or negative transformation. The technology is no longer a neutral tool.

2. The second is the *altering of a natural social behavior, or natural drive, to an unnatural dimension*, for example, when multi-player Internet gaming completely replaces person-to-person socialization (or real-life relationships). Equally of concern is when the viewing of Internet pornography, or participating in cybersex, replaces the interest or exploration

of person-to-person sexual interaction or real-life touch. The medium replaces physical human relationships.

3. The third is the *acceleration of a behavior to the realm of obsessive-compulsiveness*, for example, a health concern developing into chronic cyberchondria, or an interest in online romantic exploration developing into compulsive Internet dating. Here, usage of digital media becomes negative, or problematic, when a person continues with compulsive searching for information long after the purpose of the original quest has been fulfilled.

These three classifications are not exclusive or static behaviors or categories; they also *evolve, change, compound, and accelerate*. In summary, a loose yet rather accurate measure of when usage of digital media becomes problematic is 1) when one can't do without, 2) when one can't stop, 3) when one chooses an Internet or i-tech activity consistently over all others, and finally, 4) when there is some form of dismissed, or ignored, repercussion, or consequence, interpersonally, scholastically, or professionally. In other words, quite simply, when the usage starts to have the properties of addiction.

CHAPTER TWO

The Pull

So far I have written briefly of how digital media speeds up our brains, making it harder to find states of quiet or repose. I have also brought up positive and neutral adaptation, or what I refer to as healthy integration, versus negative interference. Regardless of what may or may not be going on in our personal and work lives, however, most of us are pulled into the medium. Why?

Process

It's all about process. Quite simply, the process of the medium, of i-tech itself, is what is attractive; it draws us in. And this draw, or pull effect, is what has the potential to alter behavior. This is not new; process itself has long been implicated in the development of certain forms of addiction. For example, the central concept in behavioral addiction, as opposed to substance addiction, is that the lure actually has very little to do with outcome. Rather, it is the intrigue, "the high," offered by the procedure itself. Think gambling.

Identical to the gambling process, digital or i-media functions on a variable reinforcement schedule. The frequency and saliency of searches and communication are random.[11] [12] Translation out of science-speak, what this means is we cannot predict the outcome or, in gambling language, the reward level of a search, message, or move. And it is precisely this, the unpredictability, that draws us in.

When a response (or reward pattern) is unpredictable or random, we are intrigued not only by *what* we might find, but *if* we will find it, and *what* quality, and *what* quantity, and *if* there is more, and *if* it will be better, etc., etc. This is "the process" that makes us want to click on items or push the "enter" or "send" button again and again; the process entices us.

Quite simply, we get caught in a loop of wanting to find out what we will see and what will happen. We continue pushing said "enter," "send," "search," and the "on" or "off" button because of the potential of reward and the mini adrenaline thrill of the unknown. It is much more than mere curiosity; we actually become somewhat high on the mini shot of anticipation (and not necessarily the result per se).

Again, just as in gambling, most of us do not stop when we win the desired sum, or find what we initially wanted. We continue wanting "it," the reward. We want more of "that feeling."

All About Anticipation

In digital media, it is the anticipation within the pause before the next Skype or text response pops up, or the anticipation of the potential that the next profile will be that of the more perfect man on a dating site, or that the washing machine at the next store online will be 10% less, that keeps us engaged. It is the magic combination of the thrill of both process and content, and it never closes. The net is always open, always accessible, anywhere, anytime, 24/7.

The phenomenon is not new at all, nor is its ability to keep us engaged. Indeed, casinos figured this out long ago. They make more money by being open all the time and keeping us guessing with both the variety of outcome in their games and our belief in our own strategies of play.

The Reverse Law of Limitation

In its pure form, the tension of the anticipatory state is neither healthy nor unhealthy. In fact, it often is great fun, but it can twist rather quickly when presented without limitation(s).

In an old world analogy, it is the brain state of the moment a person is presented with a wrapped gift, and the mini-high they get during the unwrapping. "Is it...? Isn't it...?" We see the compounding of this brain state in full force at birthdays and gift-giving holidays, such as Christmas, with children. When multiple gifts are under the tree, the majority of children do not spend time on the unwrapped gift (no matter how much they begged for it and wanted it). They unwrap the gift, squeal with delight, and then jump immediately to the next. Most children will only go back to the gift collection once there are no more packages to be unwrapped. Some may even act disappointed there are no more. The million dollar question of the digital age is whether the expression of disappointment is due to the gift not received, or whether they just want more "highs" of the unwrapping process.

The million dollar question of the digital age is whether the expression of disappointment is due to the gift not received, or whether they just want more "highs" of the unwrapping process.

Before the days of mass marketing, off-shore manufacturing, and affluence (AKA multiple gifts), we did not have this little problem. Plainly put, this phenomenon does not exist with limited possibility (or in i-terms, limited accessibility). This state only occurs when we know there is potential for more, for better. And there is always potential for more online!

Hop for a moment to Internet dating; it is the same phenomenon.

When options are finite, for example limited to the girls at the village dance or in a university class, a young man will investigate, make a dating choice, and usually be satisfied to explore this one relationship until something goes very wrong, or a new girl shows up causing him to re-evaluate his choice. But when there are a million girls...an endless supply of Internet girls...

Unfortunately, this perception of endless possibility has far-reaching consequences, including disaffecting pair bonding, a critical component for any relationship to have any lasting success.

Neurophysiological Pleasure – What's in a High?

The unwrapping high is a very different high than the one we experience when the gift is what we wanted. The two should never be confused as they are very different brain states. The unwrapping high is that of anticipation and expectation; picture again Christmas, or rather three days before, in the minds of children.

The gift itself, in contrast, produces a state of happiness or satisfaction (or disappointment or dissatisfaction, which may also cause us to seek out more). The primary danger of the digital age is precisely that we can get trapped in the anticipation or expectation high and never become satisfied, not because we do or don't like what we received, but because there is endless potential for the high of "more." The primary danger to our health is that we are thus always "on," always searching, seeking more, never resting, never satiated, never satisfied.

This has gross social, functional, and material implications, but perhaps my greatest concern, as a practicing therapist, is the emergence of a new globalized form of brain or psychological gluttony. Set aside materialism, when any search ceases to be a quest for knowledge, or achievement, or human bonding for that matter, but rather the mere pursuit of the anticipatory high due to the effortless pursuit of "moreness," the question becomes what, if anything, will ever satiate us.

Classically, disappointment, or non-resolution, will make us move on, or continue on a quest – for more information, more knowledge, new relationships, etc. Conversely, contentment, resolution, and answers typically lead to the cessation of a specific quest; they leave us in a state of satisfaction. With i-media, increasingly, it is not disappointment or even curiosity that makes us move on; it is "more" that makes us move on. As stated above, we continue pursuing long after our original objective has been reached. The most obvious examples are online shopping, including online dating, but there are some other peculiar twists on this; take, for example, the phenomenon of cyberchondria.

In cyberchondria, individuals will search and search specific symptoms and never be satisfied by null, neutral, or positive information. The twist on cyberchondria is the "high" individuals are seeking is actually reinforced by negative, not positive, information. Thus, individuals will not end their search until they find something terribly wrong. There are many reasons for this that are specific to the digital era, including using negative information on digital platforms to gain empathy. See Dr. Rosen's work in his book *iDisorder*.[13] But the underlying phenomenon is not new; this phenomenon also exists, again, in gambling (arguably around since the beginning of humanity); in cyberchondria, as with gambling, the arousal of the disappointment, of the loss, can be higher than that of the win.

What Is Going on Beyond the High?

Beyond endless availability and endless choice, a second component feeding problematic usage, and the accompanying hyperaroused brain state, is the relationship of speed to engagement. Unlike searches in library stacks and paper encyclopedias of old, digital media is fast. We do not tire tapping on our screens to the same degree. The pacing of the medium itself keeps us aroused.

The pacing of cycles is a very important component of sustaining engagement, of becoming mesmerized or obsessed. When we know a situation is finite, or has a determined cycle, we act accordingly. Take, for example, expecting a letter, the old-fashioned way (AKA snail mail). We, of old, could get very excited about the pending arrival of a letter and we knew the mail arrived at a precise time, daily. Hence, we checked the mailbox daily. Some of us may have rushed home from school or work to check, some of us may have waited eagerly by the mailbox close to the expected delivery time. But once we determined the letter had not arrived, the cycle was complete until the next day. We may have further been sad or disappointed, but few of us obsessed on, or camped by, the mailbox overnight.

This is because we knew it was pointless; the next potential for excitement or fulfillment was tomorrow. From a brain state perspective, our brains quieted for a while, integrated the disappointment, and then slowly revved up to the next potential arrival time.

Arousal typically has a natural cycle: a beginning, some sustaining, and a positive or negative end. In healthy or normal expectation cycles, our attention can only be held so long without its known or expected reward. It can also only sustain this state so long before we become anxious, angry, and even depressed.

In healthy or normal expectation cycles, our attention can only be held so long without its known or expected reward. It can also only sustain this state so long before we become anxious, angry, and even depressed.

Another example is at a live concert. The band is late; the crowd is going wild with anticipation. But how long will the audience wait before leaving or for that matter rioting? An announcer must come on stage to either keep us engaged or keep us calm; otherwise our state changes.

Not so with digital media. Messages can, and do, arrive anytime, anywhere, and by multiple modalities (email, text,

Skype, WhatsApp, Twitter, the list is rather endless). As such, we can and do stay in states of arousal, constant states of anticipation, and yes, anxiety.

Now I'm not saying we did not do this before. When we want something, we can get a little obsessed, so obsessed that it affects our behavior, sleep cycles, appetite, etc. Take a teenage girl in the 1970s, waiting nightly by the phone for the boy she has a crush on to call and ask her to the dance...But again, usually it was a finite phase. Within a week, the boy did or did not call and accordingly the girl stopped her vigilance in either disappointment or contentment. It was a circumstantial stage, and a determined cycle.

With digital media, we can stay endlessly in heightened arousal or anticipatory phases. In a new twist, we can (and do) also instigate or create the environment, the circumstance for our own arousal. We can create, or cause, our own mini-highs, our own anticipatory "unwrappings" by leaving our phones, computers, or other i-devices on. We further can up the ante by going "fishing"; we send emails and texts or even, in the extreme, troll, creating the environment for the mini-high, awaiting the response(s) to our inflammatory comments. Look at the patterns in liking and not liking on Facebook, posting and voting on selfies, starting e-rumors, posting subtly provocative comments and, obviously, Twitter. For all postings, we await, we want, we expect response.

Secondary Costs

A secondary caveat of hyper-arousal is its effect on judgment. Elevated speed and engagement limit opportunity for distraction, and critically, they do not allow for the quiet time required for processing or integration of information or related emotions. How many teenagers and celebrities have gotten themselves in massive trouble not thinking before posting or tweeting? (How many have drawn great attention to themselves intentionally doing the same?)

Again, think gambling, and games at fairgrounds. The speed

and the flash of the cards or the wheel, or the banter, and the lights are what keeps us engaged. These are what mesmerize us and lock us in. For most of us, if we have pause-time to think, we can, and do, eventually disengage. We think on our own and, in the pause, we frequently move on to other things.

The street entertainer loses some of his audience when he changes instruments or does a costume change. The politician loses some of her undecided audience with an intermittent microphone failure. Digital media, by the nature of the mechanism itself, however, does not pause on its own; it continues to flash, to pop up, to offer similar content, entice with more. When a site fails, or loads too slowly, there is always the option to instantly click on something else, to move on to the next page or i-instrument without pause. With i-tech, we actively have to remove ourselves, or, perhaps more accurately, turn our devices off.

A second component here has larger implications for education, partnering, and parenting. Both the content and the pacing of digital media keep our brains revving very fast; they keep us in said "high," and, when we are high, or getting high, we do not want to be interrupted. We do not want the sensation broken. Accordingly we abreact: get angry or upset at those who distract us. We want to enjoy this sensation. We act like addicts.

It Is the Medium Itself...

At the onset of the phenomenon, one scholar, Shaffer, stated that it was the technology itself that was the cause of our "addictive" behaviors.[14] The technology initiated, expedited, and thereafter sustained them. Shaffer further claimed that the increase in the prevalence of problematic behavior was due to an increase in accessibility of personal computers. He felt opportunities to engage in activities, in turn, were associated with higher potential for addiction and that problems were becoming increasingly prevalent due to widespread access of the Internet.

Surely, ease of accessibility, including the medium not presenting situational (e.g., location) or functional (e.g., financial) inhibitors, as well as the specific ability to cater to the precise needs or desires of the individual, is what renders i-media highly addictive. It is the perfect storm.

For many, however, the technology is effectively applied for benefit or pleasure in work, scholastics, social communication, and entertainment, and never crosses the line. Yes, we are intrigued by, and partake in, the pull (e.g., texting, searching, gaming, etc.) but we do not succumb to it. This raises a central question: apart from budding psychosocial difficulties, as most likely in the tale of Jeff and Steve, what are the features or factors that make one individual succumb to the process, even to an addiction, and another not? Why does one young woman obsess over her iPhone in all contexts while another can put it down and enjoy a romantic evening with her boyfriend, checking, but intermittently, as true to modern times?

CHAPTER THREE

The Biological Science: What's Really Going On in Our Brains?

Measuring Systems and Personal Brain Wiring

In previous chapters, I have talked about emergent history: the subtle and not so subtle cultural and personal shifts occurring with the introduction of i-tech. I have also introduced the notion of integration versus interference of i-media in our personal and professional lives. With this I have pointed out some red flags in our own behaviors and few guidelines to help one determine if usage is likely to become problematic, or not. Lastly, I introduced some of the phenomena behind the allure: the melding of physiological process with technological process.

In this chapter, I am going to get down to the hard science: what really goes on in our brains when we over-engage in i-tech. To this end, I will introduce modalities that permit us to examine the i-phenomenon at a neurological level. I will also explore the research on the alliance of i-technologies and severe brain deregulation and mental illness, AKA how under the right, or perhaps more aptly, wrong, circumstances, intrigue, anxiety, and anticipatory states can turn into true-blue pathology.

A Unique Period in History

Post industrial revolution, digital media may be referred to as the second wave of mass modern change. After television, it is possible that no other innovation within the past fifty years has changed the way we think, act, and interact with equivalent impact. Unlike the innovations that came before, however, digital media has evolved in an era that has tools to specifically examine the medium's effect on brain function and brain development.

For those of us involved in specific fields of psychology and neuroscience, this makes for an exciting era. Specific to my modality of research and practice, neurotherapy and electroencephalography, we have clear *normative* and *clinical values* of brain function from before our assimilation of the medium. What this means is that we have data on brain efficiency and inefficiency from before our full cultural immersion in digital technology. This, in turn, allows us to concretely observe and calculate the progression of the effects of the digital era on our brains.

We can now tangibly examine how digital media is changing the way we think and act on a biological, not just a social, level. We can see how our brains are modifying. We can see more than just cultural or societal (AKA behavioral) observations as discussed in the previous chapters: we can see changes in neurobiological process.

Normative Values: The "normal" or efficient brain function. Measurements of brain activity of people who have no reported or diagnosed psychological or psychosocial issues (including learning, behavior, mood, addiction, etc.).

Clinical Values: The variant or inefficient brain function. Measurements of brain activity of people with active symptoms and diagnosis of psychological or psychosocial issues (e.g., ADHD, depression, anxiety, addiction, psychosis, etc.).

When normative and clinical values are compared and contrasted, we have concrete (specific) parameters that relate to brain efficiency and health versus brain inefficiency and symptomatic states, traits, and behavior associated with specific ailments, disorders, and in its extreme, pathology.

This is truly unique. Although we may have socially observed many of the psychological and psychosocial effects of preceding technologies, we do not have solid before and after neurological measures for them; we do not have the untainted scientific quantifier or what we call pre-post evidence.

Take again, for example, television. In the case of TV, we definitely noted its mesmerizing brain and body effects. The cultural evidence is clear. Look at our older metaphors and nicknames for ourselves and the device itself: "couch potato" and the "boob tube." We also studied it and wrote about it rather thoroughly.[15] But despite scientific observations of compromised processing abilities and cultural observations of its sedentary effects, we do not have equivalent inter-generational pre-post data of brain activity on the effects of TV that are not arguably culturally biased. We have data from communities with or without TV as opposed to a world or generation before and after TV.

The historical timing of the emergence of digital technology within the era of brain mapping provides us with concrete insights as to how the Internet, including all digital media, is actively changing brain function and processing. I also have strong preliminary evidence that the medium (i-tech) is more than temporarily altering states that regulate behavior, such as social interaction and thinking. In the very young, it appears it may be changing brain development itself.

I also have strong preliminary evidence that the medium (i-tech) is more than temporarily altering states that regulate behavior, such as social interaction and thinking. In the very young, it appears it may be changing brain development itself.

The Merging of Biological Science and Social Science: How We Measure Brain Function

As mentioned in the introduction to this chapter, we are blessed to be living in an era that can accurately measure brain function, including the effect and draw of substances or behaviors on brain process. Electroencephalography (EEG) is one such method that can tell us a lot. It is the principal modality I use in both clinical practice and clinical research.

Electroencephalography 101

Electroencephalography, otherwise referred to as EEG brain mapping, or simply EEG, is a complex neurological measurement system. It is a non-invasive procedure that reads electrical patterns measured in hertz (Hz) from the upper layer of brain matter (the cortex) via electrodes placed at precise locations on the scalp (based on the international 10/20 placement system). The electroencephalographic or EEG patterns are called brainwaves. Brainwaves can be read "raw" by variation in systematic patterns or morphology (shape). They can also be neurometrically converted and read by amplitude and ratios (numbers).

EEG is a branch of brain mapping that shows how an individual's brain is working and in what degrees (e.g., extremely efficiently to very inefficiently). It is different than other mapping techniques (e.g., fMRI and PET) as the readings tell us how the brain is actually functioning (electrically) rather than show us variations in brain structure or blood flow that imply function.

By clinical standards, EEG readings can be rather precise. For example, readings can differentiate between focus difficulties due to under-stimulation, over-stimulation, and excessive challenge: three "brain causes" of ADHD that have very different underlying functional or biological mechanisms (brain states) as well as different regional sources (locations of brain deregulation) that are all associated with a set of fairly identical symptoms in a specific learning disability.

In general, EEG readings show electrical patterns (by relative amplitudes and ratios) associated with positive, negative, and normative states and traits of a person. For example, the readings show patterns associated with drive, intelligence, creativity, cognitive flexibility, emotional balance, and potential for superior numerical processing abilities. They can also show anxious or hyper states, as well as predisposition to depression, self-medicating behavior or addiction, and attention difficulties.

In the positive realm, EEG variations can show us potential for great creativity and innovation. In the negative, the variations tell us about the severity or degree of symptoms of pre-existing disorders. For example, depending how far off an EEG reading is from normative AKA "normal," a reading can show us how severe a person's depression is, or how anxious an individual may feel. The readings can also speak to liability.

TABLE 1.

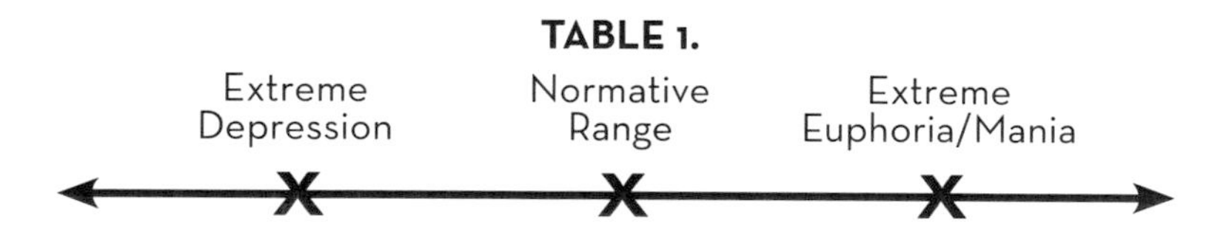

It is extremely important to note that liability refers to potential, not to fact. For example, an EEG reading may reveal that an individual's brain is inefficient in processing stress, but it does not mean this individual has an anxiety disorder. This latter quantification is most critical. Plainly put, just because you have a liability indicated by the EEG does not mean you have, or will develop, a disorder. It means you have a liability, if or when things go wrong.

Liability: What the Brain Prone to i-Addiction Looks Like

What I have discovered in my EEG research on i-addiction is that neurological liability is central to the development of excessive or detrimental Internet or i-tech usage. Any non-normative neurometric variation (EEG numbers that indicate patterns are not standard) in the EEG is a liability. Referencing Jeff and Steve again, something probably was not quite right with Jeff, whereas Steve was probably neurophysiologically balanced.

In one of my studies, I found that 77% of individuals diagnosed with an Internet Addiction had a significant EEG deregulation.[16] And I mean significant. (*For those of you familiar with the bell curve and statistics, my criterion for inclusion was a z score of plus or minus 2.*)

The simple implication of my study is: if any part of brain function, whatsoever, is significantly "off," an individual is susceptible to developing a problem. A good analogy may be the immune system. If an individual's immune system is weak or compromised, through pre-existing illness, fatigue, stress, or poor nutrition, he or she is considerably more liable to other illness, be it a cold, the flu, or more severe conditions such as pneumonia or opportune viruses such as those believed to cause Bell's palsy.

In this same study, I also confirmed that specific brainwave patterns or clusters (otherwise known as EEG signatures or phenotypes), associated with depression, anxiety, emotional deregulation, ADHD, and perseveration, are strongly implicated.

All, as in 100%, of participants in my study showed a clinical EEG signature associated with anxiety/agitation, insomnia, and addiction; 89% showed a form of ADHD (high frontal Alpha brainwave ADHD); 66% showed a signature associated with compulsive perseveration/fretting or Obsessive Compulsive Disorder (OCD); 40% showed imbalanced frontal lobes associated with emotional deregulation (typically depression); and 27% showed a signature of deregulation in the Sensory Motor Rhythm (SMR) associated with lack of bodily or physical stillness and

I believe that this liability is the key to why some of us succumb to the negative influences of digital media while others do not...

lack of focus, again associated with specific forms of ADHD. (I did not look at any patterns that were evident in less than 25% of the participants.)

I believe that this liability is the key to why some of us succumb to the negative influences of digital media while others do not: in sum, individuals with these brainwave patterns or clusters are highly susceptible to this new form of addiction.

TABLE 2.

Percentage of the Sample Meeting Criterion of Clinical Data Base Symptom Cluster	% of Sample
Anxiety/Agitation, (Insomnia) & Addiction	100%
High Frontal Alpha ADHD	89%
Compulsive Perseveration/Fretting & Obsessive Compulsive Disorder	66%
Emotional Deregulation	40 %
Lack of Bodily or Physical Stillness & Associated Lack of Focus	27%

Liability by itself, however, is not enough; it is not in itself a sufficient cause of addiction. As we know from the field of epigenetics, inherited genes or allele sequences are not always indicative of the absolute development of many diseases or disorders. For most conditions to manifest, the liability (genotype or phenotype) needs a turnkey to express itself.[17]

If I lost anyone here, this is just a rather fancy way (AKA science-speak) of saying you need two ingredients to make a cocktail. First, you need a liability allele or gene (or in my language, a liability EEG phenotype) as opposed to a protective or resilient one. Second, you need an environmental trigger (e.g., parental abandonment) as opposed to an environmental buffer (e.g., a supportive older sibling). In essence, you need both a biological liability *and* a social/environmental spark. Back to analogies, alcohol will not ignite without a match.

CAUTIONS

A point to be repeated incessantly throughout this book is that even for those with determined liability or those neurologically "at risk," digital media in itself is not negative. Continuing with the alcohol analogy, similar to individuals with significant patterns of alcoholism in their families, the inherited allele (genetic marker) is not the absolute predictor of developing alcoholism. Repeatedly, addiction research concludes, succumbing to an addiction is directly correlated with having the allele (genetic liability) *and* the inability to escape or effectively manage family discord. There are also many extreme alcoholics who do not have genetic liability: between 45 to 55% in fact.[18]

> ...any unchecked overconsumption of *any* substance, including digital or i-media, can become problematic, regardless of protective or vulnerable genetic inheritance.

For those of you now totally confused, a good way to think about this is: any unchecked overconsumption of *any* substance, including digital or i-media, can become problematic, regardless of protective or vulnerable genetic inheritance. Back to alcohol analogies: just as alcohol is a lovely substance leisurely consumed with friends, family, and food for some of us, for others it becomes a mood-altering substance that ruins self, relationships, functionality, and in its extreme even causes death. Over-consumption or misuse of digital media has the same capacity to turn bad – but it needs help.

This is not dissimilar to what much of cutting edge medicine and psychology are saying today in regards to all illness: it is the interplay of genetics and environment that determines the emergence or resistance to any specific disorder.[19] [20] [21] [22] The interaction of the genotype with the environment either protects or increases vulnerability to anything.

Negative, positive, and neutral outcome of i-tech usage appears to be directly dependent upon the interaction of our base neurophysiology (or genetic liability) with our ability to manage our physical and social environment(s).

So What's Up When Things Really Go Wrong: Pathological Usage and i-Addiction

The Big 3

So now that we know about liability and environmental triggers, what's up in the most severe cases? How and why does true i-addiction develop? How does an individual transfer from liability – to somewhat excessive usage – to actual pathological usage or mental illness? Enter the "big 3": anxiety, depression, and obsessive-compulsive disorders.

Agreement

Scholars, researchers, active practitioners, and great conversationalists tend to challenge each other, often disagreeing. It is a great part of what drives knowledge and makes the exploration of the hard and soft sciences so fun. Out of geek circles, however, disagreement is also one of the critical components that advance science itself. That said, every once in a while there is complete agreement. Currently, in the field of i-addiction, unequivocally, the heavy hitters (not those sponsored by outside interests) agree.

What has been found universally in research on problematic Internet usage, including my own, is for individuals who become complete i-addicts, those who fall off the cliff so to speak, there is a concrete relationship between anxiety, depression, and the obsessive-compulsive spectrum (including ADHD). But why? Why are these disorders so aligned with excessive usage patterns?

Getting Drawn In

As hinted in previous chapters, it all boils down to the "why" and the "how": why people use i-tech and how people use i-tech. The answer comes rather unanimously from multiple sources. Research on i-addiction has found that for adults, youth, and teens, Internet activity is frequently a direct means used to escape real life problems (the environmental trigger spoken of above). These are most commonly family discord, loneliness, and guilt. The medium is also used to detract from, as well as ease, anxiety, depression, social phobias, and obsessive-compulsive disorder (the "active" liability spoken of above). [23 24]

Young and Nabuco de Abreu, in their pivotal book, speak of predictive environments, behaviors, as well as disorders associated with the excessive or compulsive usage. They found individual characteristics, co-morbid conditions, and cultural factors including environment and family dynamics all predisposed individuals to escaping to digital media.[25]

There are also common personality traits and characteristics in those who succumbed to addiction versus those who did not. In adolescence, for example, personality traits and risk factors for i-addiction are primarily depression and ADHD. In the case of ADHD, the traits include sensation seeking, impulsivity, and reduced attentiveness. In depression, they include the negative attributes of introversion such as shyness and low self-esteem. [26 27 28 29]

Paraphrasing Caplan and High,[30] the academic literature is unified in finding that psychosocial problems are directly related to the development of problematic Internet use. Rather universally, individuals with i-addiction are suffering from some other form of mental (psychological) or social (interpersonal) difficulty. [31 32 33 34 35 36 37]

In my own work, another risk factor I have found is transition. Periods of actual transition such as romantic break-ups, loss of employment, or moves, and developmental or life stage transition such as adolescence, going to university, or retirement are all critical periods where a pastime can easily turn into an addiction.[38] Individuals feeling disenfranchised, or actually belonging to a disenfranchised community (e.g., transsexuals or being gay or lesbian in a very small town) are also at significantly higher risk. One of the demographics at higher risk right now, for example, is older, newly divorced females. Kinda breaks the stereotype of the nerdy young male and the tween attached to her iPhone.

But it all makes sense. Transition is a time when many of us feel a little depressed, bored, alone, agitated, unsure. Transition is also a common bridge out of an interpersonal difficulty such as a problematic marriage, where individuals may feel a little lost.

The Devil of Dual Purpose

In the big picture of mental and physical disquiet, however, i-media serves a purpose beyond mere communication/socialization, research/information, or entertainment. To those affected with anxiety, depression, or on the compulsive spectrum, using the medium also in some form serves to mediate emotions. Here I directly speak to how and why we use the medium.

1. ANXIETY

In the case of anxiety, what anxious individuals quickly learn is that the medium gives them more control (and sometimes the sensation of full control) over situations that can cause them (more) anxiety. Usage evolves from a choice to a dependence (or addiction), as the medium indeed serves an actual secondary purpose.

Caplan and High[39] speak to how individuals with anxiety use digital media in two ways: first, to regulate against anxious mood states; and second, to mitigate against pre-existing social anxiety. Caplan[40] also explains how using digital devices as a handy tool transitions into full dependency. He found that individuals who prefer online social interaction to face-to-face interaction were at greater risk for developing problematic i-tech use. He explains how a preference quickly turns into a reliance. Individuals thereafter learn to use the medium to regulate, or alleviate, other anxiety and other affective distress. Eventually, the Internet in all forms (e.g., communication, gaming and gambling, and sexual preoccupation) starts to replace traditional, or face-to-face, support networks such as family and friends.

Using the medium in this manner inevitably leads to increased deficiencies in self-regulation (inability to manage moods). Finally, it develops into cognitive preoccupation (obsession) with the Internet itself and its compulsive use. With reliance on the medium for anxiety relief, people further become unable to detach themselves from the technology.[41] The addiction is born. Think Jeff.

As the format of the medium mitigates against social anxiety, it can also be particularly attractive to those with social inhibition or introversion. [42 43] Here, the medium can be perceived by individuals to be easier and safer than face-to-face interaction. [44] It is important not to confuse introversion with social anxiety. From my clinical perspective, there is nothing wrong per se with being a true introvert. Being quiet and quite happy in one's own company is a personality type and a lifestyle choice. There can be something wrong, however, with being an introvert and turning to digital devices as a crutch. In my professional opinion, true introverts are content being alone and, when they do socially gather, prefer small as opposed to large groups or parties. True introverts are not overly anxious or lonely; they are actually quite content in solitary activities.

There is a fundamental difference between being alone and being lonely: a difference that often gets blurred under the title of introversion. In contrast to what I refer to as true or healthy introverts, pseudo introverts feel lonely and isolated and are often terribly anxious when in groups. They are seeking a mechanism to reach out. Enter digital screens. In this arena, Davis, Flett, and Besser[45] found that anonymity and the shield of the screen (when compared to face-to-face interaction) decreased self-consciousness, thus making it a functional mechanism for those with social anxiety.

The medium is also particularly attractive to individuals with intimacy issues or intimacy disorders. This is because all communicative interactions can be technologically mitigated. A digital device allows an individual to precisely control timing (responding, not responding, pausing, delaying response) of information as well as the quantity (what and how much to share and not share) of information. Thus, intimacy can be precisely controlled. [46 47] It is all about control of the "what" and the "when."

Using the medium as a control mechanism or mood regulator, however, is very highly associated with negative outcome. When used in this manner, it most commonly results in interpersonal difficulties at home and at work, again supporting the thesis of the multiple writings of Caplan previously referenced.

This goes far beyond social anxiety to all forms of disquiet, regardless of source. i-media is also an ideal tool of avoidance: the perfect place or activity in which to hide (or procrastinate). For those who are anxious because of perceived under-stimulation (bored or don't know what to do with themselves), it is also the perfect place or tool to keep busy, to stay occupied (stimming or staying active to calm). In essence, it is pure self-medicating.

On the EEG, the anxious profile looks identical to the addiction signature (cocaine, sex, alcohol, eating disorders, you name it). It is an elevated fast to slow brainwave ratio; or low Theta/Beta brainwave ratio (below 1.8) in the back of the brain (the occiput). In the back of the brain, the job of slow waves is to quiet. With anxiety, the EEG profile is upside down: having far too much of the fast (alert or stimulating) wavelengths and not enough power in the slow (quieting) wavelengths to counter it for balance, hence why this overactive brain type seeks stimulation to quiet. If you are having trouble grasping this concept, think of the pharmaceutical approach to hyperactive ADHD. We give hyperactive children a stimulant (typically methylphenidate) to quiet them. We stimulate this brain type more, to satisfy its higher need (for stimulation). It needs more, not less, stimulation to be satisfied to quiet, to calm.

2. DEPRESSION

I have already touched on mood and mood regulation when speaking about anxiety. Depression, however, looks quite different from anxiety on the brain in the EEG. Depression is marked by a frontal cross-hemispheric disparity in any EEG bandwidth (Theta, Alpha, and Beta brainwaves). What this translates to is if the left frontal lobe of your brain is not electrically balanced with the right frontal lobe of your brain, chances are you are less emotionally balanced and your brain is less emotionally regulated. With such an imbalance, one is prone to developing depression, and other forms of emotional volatility such as deficient anger management skills and other behaviors that can lead to interpersonal difficulties.

In the field of electroencephalography, from research, practice, and clinical data bases we have determined that any difference in electrical amplitude (*electric signal strength*) between the left frontal lobe and the right frontal lobe exceeding 15% is highly associated with mood deregulation.[48] The bandwidth electrical frequency (Theta, Alpha & Beta brainwaves) and left or right dominancy (*is left stronger than right or vice versa?*) also give us further information. Reactive depression (*e.g., mourning*) and hypervigilant depression (*e.g., feeling unsafe*), for example, look quite different than genetic depression (*e.g., blue moods and negativity running in the family, regardless of hardship and life circumstance*).[49 50 51 52]

Specific to depression and internet addiction research, there are a couple of key findings in the literature. First, depression is viewed as both a predictor and a co-morbidity of i-tech addiction; it is explored as a cause, as well as a symptom. Studies indicate that individuals with mood deregulation can be drawn to excessive i-tech use, or in contrast, mood deregulation can develop due to excessive i-tech use. In summary, the relationship of depression to i-tech addiction appears to go both ways.[53 54 55]

From the perspective of one who works in the field of EEG, this makes perfect sense. I have found all forms of frequency disparity between the left and right frontal brain lobes in both clients and research participants who identify with having i-addiction (*all kinds of stronger and weaker brainwave patterns in the left versus right side of the front of the brain*). This implies there are all kinds of causes for, or types of, depression. With these findings, it seems perfectly natural that individuals would fall into excessive Internet or i-tech usage patterns because they are not feeling well or, conversely, that they start feeling unwell due to the isolation of excessive usage.

Regardless of the chicken and egg dilemma, depression is consistently described as a vulnerability factor in all age groups. [56] [57] In a survey of over 4,000 Massively Multiplayer Online (MMO) game players, Caplan, Williams, and Lee found that loneliness was the "single most predictive factor" (p. 1319) for problematic Internet use.[58] Just as with anxiety, seeking this medium to fulfill social needs temporarily alleviates the (negative or loneliness) sentiment but then leads to additional aggravation of the original emotion. In sum, bingeing online may make one feel better for a moment but then it makes the emotion considerably worse. Caplan et al. further found that external life factors (again, the environmental trigger) were the driving factor behind problematic use.

Scientific Corner: From the pharmaceutical as opposed to EEG perspective, studies, notably Bostwick and Bucci (2008)[59] and Dell'Osso et al. (2008),[60] found the use of antidepressants successful in either eliminating or significantly reducing addictive behavior on digital media. This implies that either IA responds to the same treatment (has the same neurochemical mechanisms) as depression or is a behavioral manifestation of depression. In sexually impulsive behavior and paraphilia (such as cybersex and excessive pornography consumption), the co-morbid rate of mood disorders with IA is 70% (Raymond, Coleman, and Miner, 2003[61]). In accordance, SSRIs, SNRIs, and opiate blockers (antidepressants and pain medications) have been found effective with severe cybersex compulsivity (Kafka, 2000;[62] Karim, 2009;[63] Raymond, Grant, Kim, and Coleman, 2002[64]).

---

3. OBSESSIVE COMPULSIVE DISORDERS AND IMPULSE CONTROL DISORDERS INCLUDING ADHD

A discussion that is gaining force in the academic literature is whether i-addiction is an addiction unto itself or a perfect overlap of compulsive, impulsive, and addictive behavior.[65]

Looking from the perspective of the EEG, the overlap position again makes complete sense. As outlined earlier, my research also showed what we refer to as a cluster pattern (a grouping of liability signatures on the brain). No surprise, the cluster is in keeping with the general discussion of a perfect overlap of disorders, or what we call co-occurring disorders. (The signature for anxiety/addiction 100% is overlapping with the signature for perseveration/OCD 66%, which is overlapping with one form of ADHD 89%, and another form of ADHD 27% of the time.)

Many researchers, practitioners, and scholars are now starting to view i-addiction as they view all addiction. That is, addiction, by definition, is a problem involving impulse control regulation and an obsessive-compulsive behavior, and so too i-addiction.

Scientific Corner: Fontenelle et al.[66] discuss how OCD, and ICDs (including ADHD) and substance-related disorders, have very high co-morbid rates, share common variation in neurochemistry and neurocircuitry, neurocognition, phenomenology, as well as family factors (again the magic combination of genetic liability and environmental trigger). Pies (2009)[67] also questions if IA is "a manifestation of an underlying disorder or a discrete disease entity" (p. 31). Pies notes the blurring of definitions of addictions and compulsive behaviors and explores the literature questioning the phenomenon of IA. He discusses IA as a secondary manifestation of specific disorders such as depression and personality disorder(s). He queries whether IA is a manifestation of symptoms of other disorders including psychosocial problems that have found a home, or an expression, in a new medium. In sum, i-addiction is a behavioral manifestation of another disorder.

te Wildt et al. (2010),[68] in a similar exploration, examine IA as an independent addiction, as an impulse disorder, as well as a symptom of another disorder. They conclude that the Internet had potential to become an addiction for individuals with subclinical pathologies (disorders that were present, but not quite strong enough for diagnosis).

Dell'Osso, Marazziti, Hollander, and Altamura (2007)[69] classify IA as a newer Impulse Control Disorder. They place the disorder in the same category as Skin Picking, Tricotillomania, Pathological Gambling, Pyromania, Intermittent Explosive Disorder, and Compulsive Buying. They support a consistent relationship in earlier literature between ICDs and the Obsessive Compulsive spectrum. While the literature is in agreement regarding the relationship of ICDs including OCD to IA, studies have found varying degrees of association and co-morbidity. For example, in a study exploring the psychiatric features of problematic Internet usage, Shapira, Goldsmith, Keck, Kohosia, and McElroy (2000)[70] found that in their sample of 20 individuals, all 20 met the DSM-IV criterion for OCD as per the Yale-Brown Obsessive-Compulsive Scale. In contrast, in a sample of 16 (males and females) exploring clinical features and psychiatric co-morbidity of compulsive computer use, Black, Belsare, and Schlosser (1999)[71] found 10% of their sample met the criterion for OCD. Measures used were the Diagnostic Interview Schedule, the Minnesota Impulsive Disorders Interview, and the Personality Diagnostic Questionnaire-Revised. Bernardi and Palanti (2008)[72] examined clinical features and co-morbidities in a study on detachment and dissociative symptoms in IA. They found 7% of their sample (of nine females and six males) met the criterion for Compulsive Personality Disorder. They further found a direct correlation between higher scores on the

Yale-Brown Obsessive Compulsive Severity and the severity of IA as per the Internet Addiction Scale.

The variation in findings regarding both the frequency of co-morbidity and strength of the relationship of IA with the Obsessive-Compulsive spectrum is quite possibly directly related to Bernardi and Palanti's (2008) findings that the severity of IA is correlated to OCD or vice versa. This perspective may also be extended to depression. As found by Caplan, Williams, and Lee (2009),[73] the more severe the loneliness (depression), the more likely the individual is to be drawn to the medium in an attempt to alleviate the underlying emotion leading to problematic use and, potentially, IA.

So, is IA a discrete disorder, a behavioral manifestation of another disorder, or acceleration of a pre-existing, or subclinical, pathology? Higher rates of specific co-morbid and co-occurring pathology with IA imply that the medium (digital technology) is merely the method by which a specific pathology, such as anxiety disorder or depression can manifest. If so, IA then follows the self-medication model wherein an individual initially engages in the addiction to alleviate a specific symptom of a specific ailment (e.g., to temporarily relieve loneliness in subclinical depression through multiplayer gaming, or to relieve angst in an anxiety disorder through the viewing of pornography). The behavior evolves into an addiction as the individual is thereafter driven to the behavior regardless of negative outcome.

But If We Are Not Addicted or Otherwise Unwell, Why the Concern?

Indeed, even though we may have liabilities, we are not all addicted or suffering. So, apart from curiosity, and our own education on the i-addiction phenomenon, why should we be concerned? Many professionals and scholars hold this position. Others acknowledge liability and qualify that this is not new: stating that i-tech presents risk for addiction as did any other innovation which came before, and those which will come after.[74] With any new technology, some of us are at higher risk. We should expect no different with i-tech; some of us, the liable or the weaker, will fall prey, always have, always will. I agree with this general thesis; however, in difference to yesteryear, I believe today the stakes are higher. i-technologies and their effect on us are notably different. The instant, uninterrupted, and unlimited accessibility of both activity and content that i-tech provides is significantly changing the big picture, not only isolated frames.

When I was a teenager, indeed we did have pre-tech addicts, notably pinball followed by arcade addicts, many dysfunctionally so. But nothing that approached the level and mere volume of people affected today. Again, it is the availability, the access issue. Pre-Internet the phenomenon affected a select portion of the population. Today i-tech is affecting us all.

That said, it is affecting us to significantly different degrees, and for different reasons. I have explored some of the mental reasons but what of the cultural? What are the larger political and cultural factors behind the i-tech explosion? In the next few chapters I will address precisely this, the cultural factors that have permitted i-tech to find its niche. As always, some most positive, and some less.

CHAPTER FOUR

Boxed In: Anxiety in the Masses

So now that we know about i-addiction and i-addicts, what about the rest of us? We are not all running around anxious, obsessed, or depressed...are we?

As discussed in Chapter Two, the second caveat of always being plugged in is its effect on arousal. We are now always on: hovering over i-devices, attention divided, multitasking. Many voices state that the young are adapting quite well in such states of hyper-functionality. This is their world. It is the older individual, the digital immigrant, that can't cope. In sum, we are wired the old way and indeed are not as functional in the new digital world. We, as well as our brains, have not evolved in, nor adapted to, parallel functioning as have digital natives. Few of us can listen to music and focus effectively. We can't have two simultaneous conversations: one face-to-face and one texting. But just because *we* can't does not mean *they* can't. Hence we should get off our high horses and stop judging, stop pontificating.

Perhaps, but I would like to keep the debate open, explore what else is happening, specifically, what is happening in our neurophysiology: in our brains and our behavior when living, or rather operating, from the higher states of arousal necessary for such dual brain function. There appears to be a very strong connection between higher (and sustained) functional arousal and higher anxiety. I would also like to stay on theme: this is not all due to i-tech. Apart from technological advancement itself, many larger cultural factors at play have permitted i-tech to find its particular niche in our lives.

Revved Up and Stressed Out

Anxiety and its little buddy stress are on the rise in adults and, most troubling, increasingly also in children, adolescents, and youth. As mentioned in earlier chapters, clinically, we are all now consistently revving at much, much, higher levels. It appears all of us are functioning in significantly higher states of arousal. Accordingly, the rates of anxious depression, anxiety, and insomnia are skyrocketing as can be seen by pharmaceutical sales and rates of prevalence in the general population.

At the clinic where I practice, intake brainmaps universally reflect these higher levels of arousal. In all clients, we are systematically seeing the EEG or brainwave markers for liability to anxiety and the ability to self-quiet drop (*remember this is reversed, you want them higher as a protective factor*). Accordingly, we are also having increasing numbers of people report extreme anxiety, insomnia, behavioral and substance addictions, and just plain fretting. Ten years ago, a Theta/Beta ratio under 1.80 in the occiput (back of the brain) would indicate an individual is liable to conditions mediated by hyper- or over-arousal. It still does, but now we are systematically seeing 1.00, .90, and yes even .50. This is virtually a non-functional state of arousal: a state of arousal that a person can definitely not maintain without developing serious burnout, adrenal fatigue, depression, and of course severe anxiety itself.

Same for children: ten years ago extreme anxiety was a relative rarity. Its cause, just as with adults, was overt and insupportable life circumstances or genetically based neurological deregulation in brainwaves in areas of the brain governing perseveration and emotional regulation (*asymmetry in the frontal lobes and elevated Gamma*).

Now I see children for anxiety on a daily basis, and the anomalies are currently in the occiput, the back of the brain, again the region responsible for the inability to self-quiet. Same as their elders, little children too are in high states of arousal, and they cannot find their "off switch."

I also saw the occasional adolescent with an atypical inattentive ADHD profile. Here again rather than too much Theta frontally or centrally, as is classic in ADHD, the brainmap revealed not enough in the back, where its job is to quiet. For these adolescents, the inability to focus was not lack of attention at all. These adolescents were brilliant and brilliant at focus. It was sub-clinical anxiety that was overriding their ability to retain information. These were the kids who would study and then blank on the test. Or follow in class and have nothing left when asked to apply the new knowledge to an exercise thereafter. But many did not present as overly anxious. Many were externally quite composed; their brains were just revving too high. (*They are also, by the way, the children/adolescents for whom methylphenidate is often disastrous.*) I originally prided myself on discovering this non-standard anxiety-based learning disability (LD) profile: helping these kids flip with ease. But as a clinician I had to ask why. Why were we seeing more and more of these terribly anxious children and adolescents?

Two Profiles, Same Problem

Here is where the emotional-behavioral divide truly becomes apparent. In all age classifications, we are seeing more and more deregulation in areas of the brain that mitigate against, and thereafter efficiently process stress, but in two distinctly different profiles.

1. The first type of anxious person actually needs exhilaration to calm; they self-medicate with substances and behaviors or otherwise go mad. They typically drink too much, cycle, ski, skateboard, or drive too fast, and are constantly

seeking out activities to facilitate achieving states of quiet. In essence they stimulate to calm.

2. The second is afraid, fearful, trepidatious, a more stereotypical form of anxiety, one blocking performance, one that is based in the fear of doing.

Again, nothing new in the world of medicine and pharmaceuticals, hence the success of stimulants and sedatives.

So where does i-tech fit in?

The simple answer is that excessive dependency on i-tech is arousing us further, and by doing so, training our brains to rev higher. The scary one is that i-tech is conditioning us to need higher arousal to function, or should I say, want to function. The sidekick is this frequently comes with slower functional attention and of course higher anxiety. Small and Vorgan dubbed this as brain strain or techno-brain burnout causing distraction, fatigue, irritability, and depression. Not surprisingly, it also affects brain signaling. What I measure in electricity from the upper levels of the cortex of the brain (in brainwaves or EEG), others measure in hormone or chemical release and alterations in brain structure. Such studies are finding higher levels of cortisol and adrenaline as well as alterations in circuitry and structure in regions responsible for mood regulation and executive function (attention and impulsivity; namely the prefrontal cortex, amygdala and hippocampus).[75]

The scary one is that i-tech is conditioning us to need higher arousal to function, or should I say, want to function.

The Dance Between Arousal, Mastery, and Failure

i-tech, and gaming within, have a distinct role in propagating states of arousal, but so too do our personal desires and cultural expectations. A progressive theme in this book is that i-tech has a pretty strong role in our dysregulation, but so too does larger culture. One area of great influence is the current redefining of "success" and within this our expectations of ourselves.

Our expectations are now higher. We expect children to be perfectly disciplined, get A grades in primary school, and all go on to post-secondary education. We expect to excel at some art or sport, and have jobs at the managerial as opposed to the floor level. Increasingly we expect, or want, to succeed at everything. We have grown accustomed to, and now want, expect, even demand reward for mere participation rather than proof of excellence.

Enter Gaming

i-tech may have a pernicious little role in the propagation of such expectations. Indeed i-tech does reward us for mere participation. i-tech games and the way they are designed are absolutely genius. Nothing out there stimulates at the perfect rate nor has the ability to maintain engagement to the same degree. Nothing else rewards us so systematically. Gaming keeps us in very precise and very elevated arousal. The games are perfectly tiered and provide reward degree variation, reward frequency variation, and perfected progressive difficulty scales (the addictive pull spoken of in earlier chapters). In most other non-tech games, arts, or sports, at some point aptitude, skill, or dogmatic persistence comes into play in our choice to pursue. We quickly find our limitations.

i-tech games and the way they are designed are absolutely genius. Nothing out there stimulates at the perfect rate nor has the ability to maintain engagement to the same degree. Nothing else rewards us so systematically.

In other activities, few of us excel; our bodies and our brains fatigue. Our self-image or self-esteem takes a blow. In sports we fall, we reach coordination limits, we hurt ourselves, or we don't score frequently enough to maintain interest in pursuing the sport. In art we make messes, or things just don't look good. In music we screech. In sum when the reward button is not pushed frequently enough something else needs to kick in when enjoyment lessens. Something else needs to bridge us to the next skill or enjoyment level: personal desire, insistence of a parent to practice, good old-fashioned discipline, wanting to be included in a group playing a said sport, etc. And, until the advent of gaming or i-tech, something usually did fulfill this role. Otherwise, most of us would quit.

Today, some of us are: quitting, that is. Some of us are also not even bothering to play. We are playing i-games and only i-games instead; they are far more rewarding than play elsewhere, and systematically so.

For some of us, excessive use of i-tech may be training us out of training. It may also be training us out of the ability (or the desire) to sustain longer cycles toward reward or achievement. In addition to affecting formal learning, it may also be thwarting success at "play."

In my clinical practice modality, neurotherapy, when training the brain to increase its aptitude for attention in the treatment of learning disorders such as ADHD, we often use computer games ourselves. What we found very early on, however, was if we used computer screens (or games) that were too interesting or too engaging, the brain would not entrain. The child would do well on the game, but the brain itself would not become more efficient at other tasks less entertaining (e.g., school). Meaning, the games we use to teach the brain the proper state for learning, or success in general, need to be a little bit boring. Although in this book I am not really talking about neurotherapy as a clinical modality, it is most interesting to note that to learn to sustain attention we need less, not more, engaging content. None of us have difficulties sustaining attention on that which interests us.

Catch-22, 3, 4...

The first catch-22 for some of us (and in particular children), is that indirectly, i-media, due to its perfection in sustaining our attention, may be training us to quit or be disinterested in forms of play which, by their nature, require more persistence for success and reward. I also question if it is affecting the way we perceive play in general and the type of competitive play we are increasingly engaging in. Is play work? Is it fun? What is the dynamic between the two? What are the boundaries? When does practice end and play begin? When does play become work and vice versa?

Regardless of skill, digital media and gaming in general are entertaining. They are all about competition and success. Unlike other sports and games, due to perfected systems, including variation in reward cycles, they remain intriguing. Non-digital organized play, such as sports, music, and arts, has specific skill-acquiring objectives, making them simultaneously play and not play. They require systemic learning and practice to enhance enjoyment, and most have external standards by which they are judged.

For most of us, there is a lot of unrewarded practice needed to play well. Although many activities are fun, they are also work, and we may just have too much work in our lives. The effect is cumulative, when we send kids to school and then to organized activities, we are making their whole day overtly success or achievement oriented. I am the first to say that learning the pleasure of achievement (and delayed gratification) is critical. But so too is play, just plain play: laughter, silliness, horsing around...play! And i-media gives us that.

Blurred Lines – Practice and Training or Play?

In essence we may have lost the balance and blurred the lines of work and play, and i-media is in a pernicious way taking advantage of that by providing the play part. Pernicious because, in addition to the developmental cost (discussed at length in following chapters), excessive consumption of i-media ironically also reduces our ability to focus when we perceive things as tough or mundane.

Other activities do not move upwards, reward us so systematically, so successfully with such entertainment value. With other activities, we can't just hit the re-do button; when our interest wanes, we can't hit the re-stim button, switching out with the push of a finger to find something more interesting in a nanosecond. As such, i-tech and gaming change our expectation of natural gratification cycles: they deregulate them. They deregulate us.

And this is the second factor in our great attraction to i-gaming: the illusion of mastery. Gratification on demand! We feel on top of the world when we achieve a certain level or complete a game cycle, and even the most terrible of players eventually do. When such reward is almost certainly guaranteed by the structure of the format, that is an emotion we will pay millions for, and hours upon hours to maintain and feed.

The notion of delayed gratification, sticking with it to get it right, achieving true mastery to get reward, is being challenged! Bottom line, if you train the brain to high reward, that is all it will seek. No surprise, we are back to addiction. We are also on to boredom, agitation, and anxiety, and a growing prevalence of what I refer to as agitated depression.

Just as I preach that there is nothing wrong with a little i-tech, a lot wrong with a lot, so too with performance pressure. We all need a little performance pressure, but we also need a little play, pure play. I trust somewhere there is a balance between i-play and other play just as there is between other forms of work and play.

As mentioned at the very beginning of this book, we are all functioning under higher pressure with higher states of arousal: adults and children alike. Many of us have high-pressure or demanding jobs, and are increasingly selecting high-pressure leisure activities to defuse. There is a definite augment in adrenaline or competitive sport, e.g., performance-oriented cycling, dragon boating. There is also a definite augment in gaming. As part of the self-medicating model, many of us are actively seeking to maintain higher and higher states of arousal, as this is what calms us. In complete contrast there is also an augment in the practice of meditation and yoga – people needing to explicitly train to find states of calm.

So why are we still so agitated?

The catch is again due to the prevalence and pull of i-tech and its ability to sustain our interest and arousal even when partaking in non-tech activities. Once through a meditation class or a tennis match, or a glass of wine with friends, most of us immediately check our phones for text messages or events (some of us never stopped). We immediately re-plug into the system responsible for the hyper-arousal we are trying to defuse. We do not let the calm state settle. We know what we need, and we often do give it to ourselves, but then we immediately take it away. In essence, we take half of the prescribed cycle of antibiotics and then wonder why we still have the nastiest of bacterial infections.

What to Do About It

I advise clients to not immediately upset the state of exhilaration or calm they are trying to achieve though the activities they choose to engage in. I advise them to not reconnect after yoga, intense sport, or social activities, but instead to calmly walk or drive home alone, with friends or partners, without turning on digital devices – to let the state settle, to be able to experience said true exhilaration, calm, or pleasure, whatever the case may be.

Let the (arousal) cycle complete itself, allow the brain to settle into true tranquility; get the true ahhh effect. Your spouse knows you will be home at 7, you told her so this morning. Your boyfriend knows there is often traffic on the bridge and the window you arrive in is plus or minus 30 minutes, it always is. Your friend knows you are curious about her hot date; you can get the juicy details in the morning. Indeed, reconnect to the i-tech realm in the morning.

Not surprisingly, most of us cannot. The pull back to our devices is quite simply just too strong.

Rules, Rules Everywhere

Apart from the genius of an industry, and its ability to so accurately perceive what we want, need, or crave, one of the things I am consistently discussing and asking the reader to ponder is why, how, did i-tech find such a niche in our lives and in our communities? Why do we all turn to it? Good or bad, what purpose is it serving? In partial answer to this, a second cultural component is gross restriction. We are imposing structure and organization, everywhere!

We are putting children in rule-bound school followed by tightly rule-bound extracurricular activities. From a socio-developmental perspective, the pressure for success we place on little children today is ridiculous. In school, we do not let developmental stages (e.g., letter reversal) settle before we yell dyslexia. When a young one on the soccer field, karate class, art class, or choir goofs around, we complain of inattentiveness, distracting others, being off task, or good old ADHD. We are also increasingly intolerant of natural children's behavior. Little five-year-olds roll on the floor giggle and scream with delight and occasionally merely to hear the sound of their own little voices. Nothing wrong with this; it is just what kids do. But we are reacting differently. Do to our own overarousal, we are increasingly annoyed.

As we are systematically putting the pressure on discipline, we are also putting the pressure on safety. We are making helmets obligatory (everywhere, not just in hockey, BMX, mountain biking, skiing, skateboarding, or on roads with cars). We are developing swimsuits with flotation devices for beaches and swimming pools (as opposed to sticking to life jackets in boats where the danger of drowning due to accidents is imminent). We are adding elbow pads, knee pads, and braces to the vast majority of sporting activities, removing high swings, climbing ropes, and spinning platforms, lowering monkey bars, removing dirt from playgrounds and replacing it with foam... get the picture? We are systematically taking the fun, the thrill, and the adventure out of play.

The effect? When the rules get too tight, we increasingly want to break them – either for the intrigue or simply as a method of bringing back the fun. And that's just it: by over-structuring play, we take a lot of the fun out of it. Now children, just like adults, increasingly get their down time, or just plain fun time, on i-tech, and the darned medium is fun.

Brain deadening, useless, but fun...and we all need a little of that. In i-tech games no one cares if you smash the car or drive it correctly. Many games even overtly acknowledge it is considerably more fun to crash and scrape cars than to drive them responsibly. No surprise, many games are now explicitly designed to capitalize on this: overtly based on crashing rather than constructing and other forms of "fun" destruction.

From the days of Pong, Mario, and arcade racing, the industry has evolved considerably. Like any successful industry, they observe which components of their products consumers respond to and they develop them accordingly. They know what we want. They know what we crave, and they provide it. Twenty years ago we liked crashing, we liked bopping things on the head, we liked "eating" things, shooting things, and searching.

Today in response to the consumer, the gaming industry is providing more adventurous and more overtly thrilling and destructive games. And while the i-tech industry is pandering to our desires for adventure and destruction, we are systematically imposing more and more restriction in our offline lives in the name of discipline and safety.

Quite wisely, the industry is capitalizing on the fallout of our self-imposed excessive restriction; we are now looking for our thrills elsewhere and i-media is providing it. It is an obvious choice; i-media is without boundaries in a world that is closing in. To this end, the media and gaming industries are absolutely brilliant. Unlike us (e.g., many parents, politicians, educators, psychologists,

MDs, and policy makers), they are completely in tune with children's (heck, all people's) needs for such expression and exploit this increasingly unfulfillable desire for accessible thrill to market products that allow people to vent out increasingly restricted attitudes and behavior(s).[76] They got us at our own game. Our systematic intolerance for thrilling non i-media play is going against nature, human nature.

But it does not end here. We are not only systematically restricting our environment(s) and attitudes, we are also restricting our behavior. We are changing our wiring.

Restriction Part B: Thwarting the Learning of Responsibility

Perhaps more important, from a socio-developmental perspective, by trying to (over) protect ourselves, we are also taking out the need for the learning of true, or necessary responsibility: the need for the learning of boundaries of play in real life.

The child always provided with flotation devices will not be able to do handstands or submerge themselves, learning the limits of holding their breath. They will not experience the sheer exhilaration and, yes, fear of jumping or diving and then cresting above the water again in a deep lake or swimming pool, nor will they efficiently learn how to swim. In sum they will not test or learn self-sufficiency in the water, including learning not to play in the deep end when they are tired, making sure they can touch bottom when the pull of the tide is notable, or the learning/testing of fatigue limits with treading water without aid. They will not learn their limitations.

...we are also taking out the need for the learning of true, or necessary responsibility: the need for the learning of boundaries of play in real life.

Ironically, increasing protection and safety by reducing or removing the possibility of exploration of danger in play does not necessarily eliminate the desire to explore it; in fact, in the second perfect catch-22, for many, it can increase it. It can also increase the instance of actual danger and injury.

When children (and later adults) do not learn real boundaries, including appropriate respect for, and fear of, danger, the incidence of injury can and does rise. Indeed we may need more helmets, elbow pads, and flotation devices. This is part of a now notable increase in impulsive as opposed to calculated risk taking, also the increased search for more dangerous adrenaline-releasing activities. When we don't feel the danger, we seek it; we seek the missing thrill.

On the flip side of the coin, for those caught in trepidation as opposed to thrill seeking, i-tech and restriction are affecting resilience. We now rarely go far enough in non-digital play to learn through experience when we need to stop to protect ourselves, or to not harm others. We also do not learn resilience or repair. With limited exposure to boundary exploration, including potential for hurt, harm, and emotional distress in childhood, when we are actually faced with it later in life, we are defenseless. We have built no tolerance for it, no resistance; we have reduced immunity to real life.

With limited exposure to boundary exploration, including potential for hurt, harm, and emotional distress in childhood, when we are actually faced with it later in life, we are defenseless.

A population I am increasingly working with for extreme anxiety is first-year university students. Now out of the nest, and having been quite sheltered, they don't have the tools to face real life: real critiques, real expectations, or relationships unmediated by parents or guardians. As a consequence they are completely decomposing. They have never faced true failure either academically or socially and, as such, they have not learned resilience, including knowing how to repair situations and relationships, or how to emotionally repair themselves. Under such circumstances, emotional distress has a much greater effect when it does occur. Emotional stress feels like trauma as we react to lower and lower thresholds without said learned defenses.[77]

Filling Voids

You may notice I am dancing between multiple generations: children and adults. The point I wish to make is this goes for all of us, not just children. Many of us are now simultaneously bored and agitated, with lower defenses. We no longer know what to do to settle ourselves, hence the augment in anxiety, depression, and other forms of addiction. We are glued to our devices in an attempt to stay occupied, to entertain ourselves, to defer emotions. Yet by the very fact of doing so, we are feeling more agitated and void.

The Lost Art of Leisure

Until the advent of 24-hour television and i-tech, in our free time most of us used to thrive on some sort of personal expressive outlet (arts, tinkering, community games and sports, collecting, needlework, woodworking) or a solo passive outlet (e.g., reading). Prior to the second installment of modernity, or the advent of busy, busy lives, our needs were fulfilled by what we used to call hobbies.

Hobbies are considerably different from explicit maintenance activities, such as yoga or going to the gym, wherein the primary purpose is to get or keep fit or learn to reach states of mental calm. They are also different from activities that involve much comparison or competition; these factors convert hobbies to sports or to arts, or to discipline (so does obsession by the way).

Hobbies involve pure pleasure and some cognitive function as well. Many involve physical activity, strategy, or artistic expression; many also involve observation, seeking, and searching. The key difference for most, however, is they need not be, and often are not, performance oriented. Being "good" or "bad" at your hobby is absolutely irrelevant; enjoying it, being enraptured by it, is.

By definition a hobby is a leisure pursuit, a pastime, a diversion. Although some might have great high or low points, we do them because they please us, they reduce stress, reduce strain; they are directly or indirectly calming, the perfect antagonist to work or duty. The key to remember, on a neurological level, i-tech does not calm, it stimulates. Engagement does not reduce arousal at the end of its cycle; it heightens arousal. It is very, very different from a hobby in this regard.

With the exception of some card games (e.g., bridge, solitaire, and gambling games), most hobbies, particularly sport and art, need not be affected by i-media. Unfortunately one great classification of hobbying is: collecting. In collecting, many hours were spent searching, seeking, going to fairs, clubs, conferences, garage sales, trading, organizing, and researching. This can be done in an instant now with i-tech, and with i-tech it does not particularly require any skill, a special eye, or dedication (or for that matter socialization or even leaving the house). As such, reward cycles again are affected; people can find things with incredible ease online and can become dangerously obsessed with the "moreness" factor discussed earlier. Hobbies under these facilitated conditions can quickly turn into obsessions; they also become significantly more costly. Part of hobbying was budgeting; people would budget or save for "when" or "if" they found an object and then trade up or down for the more prized (in their eyes) object. It would take months, sometimes years, to find the right coin ; now you just go online and once you determine the correct sites: search, search, search, and voilà, you can buy it.

Again we are full circle back to elevated arousal, the lack of delayed gratification, and the thwarting of the true pleasures of acquisition or achievement and...moreness. Hobbies also require passion or some other emotion or drive to keep us engaged. When gratification cycles are affected, we find such activities less interesting, mundane, even boring; conversely we can also become dangerously obsessed. So much for non–i-tech hobbies...

Full Circle Back to Direction Versus Correction

We want to be very careful about what we train out in the name of discipline or safety. We also want to be very careful about what we train in. Most frequently in youth, a busy body is also the sign of a busy brain. You want to stimulate this brain, not settle it, and you definitely do not want to stimulate it with excessive i-media (see Epilogue). In this regard, i-tech should be part of the diet, not the staple. Busy brains are potentially brilliant brains and they are at higher risk of getting trapped. If a busy brain discovers easy stimulation, it will not discover creativity, from which all innovation and invention births, nor will it discover sports or arts at which it, they, will potentially excel.

Yet we ask our little ones and expect our big ones to sit still for hours on end. We keep them in from recess when they don't finish their work. We remove the fun from art, sports, and music with high expectations and over-structure. And then we ask them to be "quiet" at home and give them i-tech devices to ensure they are, as we race to prepare dinner, finish our own work, or just plop on the couch in front of the TV or our own i-devices in absolute brain or body fatigue or in our own anxiety. Of course they swallow i-tech; they gorge themselves on it and subsequently few know what to do in the absence of it. When not on it, they are bored, agitated, and so are we.

In sum, anxiety is on the rise for multiple and somewhat contradictory reasons. We are too busy, yet not busy enough. We put too much pressure on ourselves, but not the right type. We are too safety oriented, which makes us a danger to ourselves. We seek out activities to release tension and then crash, as opposed to calm naturally into healthy fatigue.

In sum, anxiety is on the rise for multiple and somewhat contradictory reasons. We are too busy, yet not busy enough. We put too much pressure on ourselves, but not the right type.

CHAPTER FIVE

From Digital Natives to i-Kids

Play, Learning, and Creativity, Part A

In previous chapters, I have spoken of risk factors and liabilities that have the potential to affect us all: young and old, those of us born into the digital age, and those of us who have migrated into it. I have also spoken of the features that render all i-media dangerously attractive and the related addictive pull. Aligned with this, I have highlighted some of the true blue factors of i-addiction: the "how" and the "why" excessive usage becomes intertwined with mental illness, some quite severe, some arguably less. I have also spoken to cultural shifts that propagate anxiety in the masses and how i-tech is not necessarily the cause but undeniably a contributor to generalized fretting and a globalized sense of disquiet many of us are now experiencing.

In this chapter I am going to speak of a critical dynamic that i-media has with play, learning, and creativity. This is a dynamic that concerns mostly digital natives, and the now very young: what I call the third generation or i-kids (what others refer to as Gen Y and Z): those who know no other world, kids born into i-tech.

Digital "Play" AKA Gaming

As a clinician, I have been long aware of the central role excessive gaming has in the development of emotional deregulation, associated trouble in interpersonal relationships, and behavioral disorders. Over the past ten years or so I have also become progressively conscious of how gaming affects cognition and learning, specifically in children. In my clinical work I have recently found something else, something that concerns me even more. It now appears excessive gaming may have a critical role in commandeering a specific brainwave associated with creativity and innovative thinking.

For those actively engaged in this gaming, however, my voice of clinical experience often falls flat. The voice of the industry promoting the benefits of gaming, educational and otherwise, is much stronger.

> It now appears excessive gaming may have a critical role in commandeering a specific brainwave associated with creativity and innovative thinking.

Parents, children, all of us, are aware of the dramatic extremes brought to us by the evening news: tragic suicides, deaths, and massacres partially attributed to excessive or obsessive gaming. But this does not relate to most of us, leaving the lesser, subtle, and compounding effects still largely ignored. In this social atmosphere, many therapists have been hard pressed to find support for their concrete clinical experience and knowledge of the research which demonstrates unequivocally that a lot of gaming is associated with many of the major and minor issues plaguing the children they are serving. Until around ten years ago, my situation was no different.

A little over ten years ago, two clients absolutely solidified my clinical concerns. They were not so extreme. These kids were not involved in the abovementioned massacres, torturing of animals, or anything that would make the evening news. Nor did they appear to be in compromised situations or from "bad" homes. They were just two young boys undeniably brought down by gaming. And it was evident in their brain deregulation. Meet Franco and Liam.

A Tale of Two Boys

Franco

Franco was a lovely, gentle, nine-year-old boy brought to our clinic for educational difficulties. He was one of those children who was a delight to work with. He was polite and quiet, and would engage when spoken to. Franco also came from a well-educated intact family. He appeared to have a good relationship with his parents and siblings. He was obviously cared for. One could tell, however, that he was a little discouraged, that the expectations of his family were high.

Franco's assessment (EEG) was unremarkable for standard attention difficulties. By clinical standards, his fast to slow brainwave activity was where it should be for efficient learning. The back of the brain was also normative, indicating no issues with agitation, self-quieting, or sleep. There were no brainwave signatures for processing difficulties or trauma. He also had what I affectionately coined as the "sweetheart signature," a brainwave pattern associated with cognitive flexibility and a personality trait of compatibility. This was topped off with a signature for superior intelligence, commonly found in adult inventors and entrepreneurs. In sum, a parent's delight.

What Franco did have, however, was a brainwave signature associated with a predisposition to depressed mood states. He also had some excessive frontal slow wave activity commonly associated with higher than average daydreaming. Not so good for school.

Scientific Corner: Summary of Franco's clinical EEG profile: Theta/Beta ratio @ Cz 2.2 that reduced with cognitive tasking (reading); Theta/Beta ratio @ O1 of 2.0 that increased in an eyes closed condition; solid Alpha response centrally and occipitally under eyes closed condition; HiBeta/Beta ratio at location Fz between .44 and .55; a low low/high Alpha ratio @ location Fz; frontal deregulation, F4>F3 Beta by 48%; elevated Delta @ Fz.

Franco was also a therapist's dream. We did a short course of treatment and Franco and his parents left delighted with his newfound ability to focus in class.

Franco, however, returned with his father six years later at the tender age of fifteen. This is not uncommon. Many former clients will return for a tune-up when they encounter a bump (e.g., a tougher class in high school or transitioning to university). Franco, however, was different. He was disengaged, grumpy, even rude – definitely significantly less sweet.

Without considering the EEG, such shifts in personality traits could be chalked up to being a teenager. At the clinic we often joke with parents regarding how the neurology can be corrected, but we can't cure adolescence. Thus, his change in presentation did not particularly concern me. What did concern me, however, was that Franco's EEG was dramatically different.

Franco's EEG now revealed the signature in the back of the brain associated with anxiety and non-restorative sleep. This signature is also indicative of a liability to addiction, something to be taken seriously in adolescence. Franco also had a signature for trauma and a different form of depression that can often manifest in expressions of anger. What had happened to this boy, now young man?

Scientific Corner: Summary of Franco's 15-year-old clinical EEG profile: Theta/Beta ratio of 1.4 @ O1 that reduced to 1.0 when he closed his eyes; Alpha brainwaves not increasing under eyes closed conditions; 20% difference in the Theta brainwave bandwidth between the left F3 and right F4 hemispheres.

One thing that is known is that trauma or exposure to extreme emotional stress can deregulate everything. And Franco's EEG was telling me that since I had seen him last he had been, or was actively in, an extremely emotionally stressful environment: a situation, or environment, he was having great difficulty processing.

Franco denied bullying, a very common cause of trauma or brain deregulation in youth, and there was no current situation or past event that his father was aware of. No death in the family, no home break-in, no pending divorce, or atypical marital strife, in essence no dramatic event that would deregulate Franco to such a degree. The dramatic shift was an enigma and so was Franco's second round of treatment. Despite working on the neurophysiology with neurotherapy, Franco did not improve as he had on the previous cycle of treatment, and I must admit I was truly stumped.

And then the bubble burst. Franco's behavioral issues had a catalyst. I soon learned that Franco was gaming hours upon hours, and that this was the constant source of strife in the household. He was arguing relentlessly with his parents when they would attempt to have him disengage from his game for chores, homework, even dinner. He was not sleeping, claiming he was not tired, and needed his game to calm. This was a new and entirely different problem.

What opened my eyes here was not that gaming was eventually identified as the problem, but rather that neither parents, nor child, had made the association of the behavioral and personality changes with the increase in gaming. Gaming was not reported or even suspected as cause. Franco's parents would report the fight but not that it occurred when or because they asked him to stop gaming and set the dinner table. They perceived the fight being over not wanting to participate in family chores, rather than not wanting to disengage from the game.

Liam

Liam was a boy of eleven. He was quite a handful. His mother reported he was defiant at school, as well as at home. He had been diagnosed with ADD, gifted learning disabled, Conduct Disorder, then Written Output Disorder, followed by Autism, and finally with Asperger's. He was on a cocktail of medications. He was completely unable to function in school, incapable of focus. He had a classroom aide as well as a personal scribe. He could not sleep; he would wake exhausted even after over ten hours in bed. He was extremely resistant to transitions and would become obsessively involved in things, would not listen or respond when engaged, and became very angry when required to stop. He had very poor peer interaction, resulting in no friends. The list on the intake form was endless. His mother was beside herself. She did not know what to do. She did not know where to turn. Both she and her child appeared miserable.

Liam's EEG was classic for ADD. This neurological profile would indeed have trouble with focus and learning. In contrast to his mother's report of chronic fatigue, however, the brainwaves associated with sleep regulation and the ability to achieve states associated with restorative sleep appeared to be good. The frontal lobes were also balanced, indicating good emotional regulation, unusual for children with reported defiance and conduct issues. What Liam did have, however, was what we refer to as a hot cingulate, which is often associated with extreme stubbornness and obsessive (compulsive) behavior and not uncommon to find in children in the autistic spectrum. Unlike Franco, Liam definitely did not have the sweetheart signature.

Scientific Corner: Summary of Liam's clinical EEG profile: Theta/Beta brainwaves @ location CZ of 3.5; Theta/Beta ratios in the occiput over 2.0 in both eyes open and eyes closed conditions; F3 = F4 in all its measures; Low/HiAlpha brainwaves of 2.25; Delta brainwave amplitude of 25 @ location Fz; HiBeta/Beta brainwave ratio .84 (normative is between .44 and .55) @ location Fz.

In complete contrast to Franco, Liam was a little devil to work with. His behavior was disproportionate to the deregulation of his brain as indicated by the EEG. He would yell and scream profanity, rip off the electrodes, and try to break the equipment. He would react to holding a pen like a vampire to garlic: holding his wrist and crying how it hurt when he wrote. He would beg his mother to massage his hand due to the pain the pen was causing, and she would comply. If this child and his mother had not been in such desperate emotional pain, the scene would have been humorous.

Fortunately I had some experience with kids like Liam. This was definitely behavioral masking and a mother who had lost control, terribly desperate for help.

Purely from an educational perspective, what kids like Liam need is help with their educational challenges, not adaptations that enable disabilities by pandering to the behavior (such as hand massages and scribes). As a general rule, if you help a child with the EEG deregulation associated with the learning challenge(s), the resistance to school and school work (e.g., writing) reduces. The defiance and the associated behavioral drama then tend to fall into place with without much further need for work on the EEG for emotional deregulation.

Authoritative strangers have an advantage with kids like Liam. We can come in with new rules of engagement and new expectations of performance and have a child comply on tasks where parents and teachers no longer can. I took full advantage of my upper hand, and within ten minutes it was perfectly obvious that Liam could write, and that indeed he had his mother and his educators completely held hostage with his outrageous behavior.

We started a behavior plan and an education plan along with the EEG work (neurotherapy) to normalize brain function. Liam started slowly turning a corner. After five months of treatment, Liam, and his mother, reported school was going well; concentration was much better and he was working independently. The aide and the scribe were soon to be out of their jobs! Things were much better in general at home as well; he was diligent about using the sleep therapy tools and reported they were really helping too. His mother further reported stress levels in the home were dramatically reduced as school work was less difficult. Liam was also no longer fighting with her about going to school. And then, progress halted and even started to reverse.

Subsequently, in my inquiry chats with Liam, I learned that Liam was gaming in most of his spare time: six to ten hours a day, he boasted. When I asked if he was exaggerating, he said "no," he does two hours of school work and chores and then all the rest of his time is on his games. "I enjoy it, my average is eight hours." I also learned that the therapy was going well in part due to an arrangement he had with his mother: that, if he complied, he could have more gaming time. I was being hoodwinked. He was being bribed. His mother was still hostage. We were back to zero.

The Significance of Gaming in Brain/EEG Deregulation

I learned much from these two boys. First, always get information upon intake regarding hours on gaming, TV, etc. Second, gain an insight into parental attitudes on gaming and digital devices. Many parents feel they are entirely innocuous. Many parents further use digital media as an aid, perceiving it as an effective and harmless tool to facilitate parenting: the perfect bribe, reward, or babysitter. Many even firmly hold to the notion that digital media including gaming is good for their children, improving processing speed, working memory, and learning in general. I don't blame them; the information parents are receiving is most confusing. And many sources are most convincing.

In the cases of both Franco and Liam, the clinical cog was indeed parental misperception or lack of awareness of the influence of gaming on the emotional heath and the learning abilities of their children. It was not brought up at intake, as the potential influence was not even considered. Franco's parents did not report that Franco's behavior started to slide with his increase in gaming. Liam's mother did not state that her comments on the intake form "resistant to transitions; becomes obsessively involved in things; does not listen or respond when engaged and becomes very angry when required to stop" was in direct reference or relationship to gaming.

My error was the assumption that parents would report excessive gaming. This oversight made me alter the structure of my intake. Upon meeting a child (and now often adults), I explicitly ask the number of hours the individual games or is otherwise engaging with i-media (and TV). Influence is now no longer limited to gaming (by the way): we see the same "invasion" and deregulation occurring with excessive digital consumption of search content and social media (Facebook, etc.). The cell phone, not the PC, is now the dominant tool of engagement. Increasingly individuals are involved in obsessive texting and checking, with a complete inability to detach. In essence, all digital media regardless of purpose or content is implicated. We have moved far beyond gaming or Internet addiction to generalized i-tech addiction.

Rising Awareness

Back to Liam and Franco: my experience was not atypical. Other clinicians and scholars reported similar experiences, and it was starting to emerge in the professional literature. In 2008, Block wrote on how excessive or disruptive i-tech usage was rarely reported at intake. Similar to my experience, he found that individuals in the US presented for the co-morbid condition (e.g., a behavioral or scholastic complaint) and, as a result, i-addiction was rarely detected.[78]

In Asia, however problems with excessive usage and i-addiction were broadly recognized, including in its extreme, beyond the media hype. There were clearly reports of a possible association of addictive Internet usage and suicides, murders, and cardio-pulmonary deaths.[79] Today, in Asia, clinics treating i-addiction are common. Mid-decade, across all cultures there was mounting evidence of a definite association with i-addiction and depression, ADHD, and suicidal ideation.[80] [81] Those in the know, namely Cooney and Morris,[82] were pushing for discussion in the clinical literature regarding the need to take an Internet history, particularly when working with adolescents and youth, again finding that excessive i-usage was frequently a compounding or a primary contributor to psychological or behavioral impairments. They, like others in the trenches, felt gaining a measure of severity of Internet usage, as well as how it affects brain function, was most relevant. In my own practice, kids like Liam and Franco were becoming more common, yet all still seeking services for the related symptom (e.g., ADHD, behavior or conduct disorders, written output disorder, reading disorder, processing disorders, dyslexia, etc.) rather than the cause or antagonist (excessive consumption of digital media). The compounding issue of i-tech misusage was still not yet on the common radar.

Fast Forward...2013–2015

Firmly ten years post Liam and Franco (and unfortunately I must say), my job is getting easier. Client or parental confirmation of excessive screen time is always helpful, but awareness and transparency are no longer critical. Clinicians are on this. We are also seeing more globalized effects. A study by Gentile in 2009[83] found that in the US 8.5% of children and adolescents (8 to 18) who game show symptoms of pathological addiction; and 88% of people in this age classification game! This is about one in ten people, and let me tell you, pathological addiction is no joke. In the study Gentile found the standard issues with education and health, but also theft to "support the habit." These are rather frightening findings, hopefully ones that will shake us out of our cultural denial. Another interesting factor is that parents were aware of the problem (but that is another chapter).

What concerns me now are the physical changes I am seeing in the brain: on the EEG. As of approximately three years ago, I started concretely seeing what I thought were functional alterations in brainwaves directly associated with excessive consumption of digital media (including gaming). This is not generalized deregulation as was apparent in Franco, Liam, as well as in my adult studies on i-addiction. It is deregulation in one specific brainwave. In positive, this is potentially a means to diagnose the problem and prove that concretely, biologically, there are changes occurring. But it is also proof that the problem now extends far past signatures associated with learning deficiencies, emotional regulation, and anxiety as seen in my clients ten to fifteen years ago. The primary brainwave I am now seeing deregulating is one directly aligned with higher function.

In the following chapter I will discuss how I discovered this and why it is of such great concern.

CHAPTER SIX

The Story of Alpha

In this chapter I will discuss my discovery of the signature for modern excess: a form of brain deregulation purely associated with excessive use of i-media. The brainwave cluster pattern referred to in earlier chapters, although common to all those with i-addiction, is not exclusive to those with i-addiction. The cluster of lack of mental and physical quiet, emotional deregulation, perseveration, and ADHD is found in other forms of pathology, including other forms of addiction. In this chapter I will introduce Alpha deregulation, a specific spindling pattern I discovered in 2012 that appears to be exclusive to the excessive or intrusive usage of i-tech.

But first, what is Alpha?

Let Go of My Alpha!

Alpha is a most unique brainwave. It really is implicated in everything: attention, intelligence, innovation, creativity, PTSD, age-related cognitive decline; the list goes on. It is also a rather finicky wave. Meaning, you want just the right amount in the right amplitude, the correct ratio, under the right condition, in the right brain location. Kind of like heart rate and blood flow variation. When you are warm or cold, exercising or at rest, excited, frightened, or calm, you want your heart and blood flow doing different things to either protect you or make you more efficient. If your body has it backwards, you can be a little deregulated or, in contrast, in some real trouble (think neuropathy, hypothermia, heart and blood pressure conditions, erectile dysfunction, etc.). Similarly when Alpha brainwaves function correctly where and when they should, you are a superstar. Think supreme professional or Olympic athletes or the greatest innovative thinkers; for me Einstein, Chomsky, and elite composers come to mind. When Alpha is not well regulated, well...neither are you.

For quite a while, I knew something was up with Alpha. But what? There was definitely some clinical connection with Alpha brainwave anomaly and excessive i-usage, but I could never quite put my finger on it. In this exploratory stage I was looking intently at the relationship of i-tech to ADHD symptoms as well as to anger, anxiety, and intelligence. And then, one day, I saw it on the EEG, and all the pieces started to fall into place.

The Alpha Connection

While cleaning EEG data for my PhD dissertation on i-addiction, I saw something very unusual. Cleaning data, or artifacting as it is technically called, involves going through the raw EEG (*brainwave patterns*) and taking out segments that are affected by movement. Eye blinks, swallows, jaw tension, and any unusual pattern (*in the raw brainwave algorithms*) attributed to movement as opposed to cortical firing (*true electrical signal or brainwaves*) are removed from the data. This can be done by computer program or by trained individuals.

In the field of EEG research, we tend to do this manually. We remove segments by visual pattern recognition as opposed to relying on a (computer) pattern recognition program. Visual artifacting by an individual trained in brainwave versus artifact morphology (*shape differences*), although long and arduous, is considered far more reliable than digital or computer-based artifacting (*computer editing*). Visual or manual artifacting is even more reliable when two trained artifactors agree on the segments to be removed.[84] [85] To this end, my colleague, Michael, graciously gave his time acting as my second artifactor. To have the data withstand any potential critique, it was further recommended by a most respected research-practitioner, Dr. Donaldson, that I submit the data for third party quantitative and qualitative reliability analysis (*tech talk for serious statistical analysis by an outside business that has no interest whatsoever in the positive or negative results*). The files received idyllic scores. My data was bullet proof. (See Appendix.)

I mention all this detail as this is where I first consistently saw this rather unique pattern of Alpha brainwaves: a pattern, I might add, that an automated computer program certainly would have deleted as the amplitude was ferociously high and it closely followed true artifact. What I saw was an eye flutter (*true artifact*), followed by very high amplitude Alpha brainwave bursts (*the real deal*). It was a very unusual pattern that, once identified, Michael and I paid special attention to. Indeed, once we were looking for it, we found it was consistent in every single EEG brainmap of every person in my i-addiction study.

Michael and I diligently removed all of the preceding eye flutters and were left with a powerful pattern of Alpha brainwaves that was *consistently* within, if not above, the parameters of an artist's signature.[86] This was telling me something quite unexpected. All of the self-proclaimed "Internet Addicts" in my study on i-addiction had innovative artistic brains!

The Joy of Alpha

So what is an artist signature in electroencephalography? The Artist Signature was first identified by Dr. P. Swingle (AKA, Dad) in the early 1990s. He discovered that when moving from an eyes open to an eyes closed condition, if Alpha brainwaves rose significantly over 30% centrally (*location Cz*), and robustly above 50% occipitally (*say above 90% or so at location O1*), it was highly correlated with creativity. This was in the modern sense of having an aptitude or interest in singing, dancing, painting, etc. It was also in the classical sense of being able to see and analyze patterns which could then manifest in a sensibility for architecture, spatial planning, musical composition, or higher levels of mathematics and the science(s).

Over the last fifteen years or so, when I saw this pattern on a child's EEG brainmap assessment at intake, I reported it to parents with delight. It was a most desirable signature, unequivocally associated with innovation, creativity, and artistry. A child blessed with this artistic signature could go far.

First Red Flags – Hijacking the Creativity Wave

At the clinic, when reporting assessment results to parents and children, we always seek out the positive or efficient brain function along with the negative or inefficient function. This is particularly important when working with children and adolescents brought in for behavioral problems or learning disabilities. These kids (and their parents) tend to be saturated with the negative. They are often very discouraged and benefit immediately from something good to hold onto beyond the ADHD, written output disorder, dyslexia, or any other neurophysiological condition for which they are seeking our psychological services. Hence, when I would see this fantastic artistic Alpha brainwave pattern, I would bring out my counter lever. "Yes, the EEG brainmap results are indeed indicative that Peter would have some difficulty with his focus in school and is perhaps a tad stubborn. But is he also innovative? Does he have artistic talent?" Consistently parents would be delighted that this not only could be seen in the brainwave patterns but that their child was validated; there were most positive components to his or her brain function too!

And then times started to change, the red flags emerging. More and more frequently parents would acknowledge that their child (typically male) had had artistic talent as a small boy but was not currently following any creative pursuits. The true punch however would come later in the course of treatment. Systematically, it would be revealed that the fading of interest in artistic pursuits occurred about the same time the child discovered video or computer gaming.

Fast forward to 2014. Whenever I see this pattern on an individual aged thirty or younger, I now query as to (excessive) usage of digital media as well as creative aptitude. I am very saddened to report that today half of these individuals never discovered the creative talent. It has been hijacked by digital media. Of note, the Alpha brainwave jump I am now seeing is becoming progressively stronger, implying more severe deregulation in more people. For those involved with excessive consumption of i-tech, it is not uncommon for me to now see Alpha rise 300% centrally and 500% in the occiput when individuals close their eyes. In this amplitude range it is also crossing over into yet another classification. Alpha spindling of this strength is what we usually associate with epilepsy, absence or catatonic seizures. What's going on?

Systematically, it would be revealed that the fading of interest in artistic pursuits occurred about the same time the child discovered video or computer gaming.

Parallel morphology of Alpha brainwaves (*seemingly identical shape and amplitude strength*) between some excessive i-tech users and individuals with catatonic seizures is my current enigma. The alarm bells are ringing but it is far too soon to draw any definite conclusions. Is this a function of overexposure to electromagnetic fields (EMF) generated from i-tech or perhaps a rewiring due to process? Who knows; but I can speak rather extensively and comfortably to the connection of gaming to innovation and creativity.

What's Going On?

Quite simply, creative or innovative Alpha is seeking a pathway for expression. And it is now finding it in gaming rather than in artistry. Similar to Theta/Beta brainwave signatures in the occiput that regulate quieting and hence speak to liability for addiction, it is merely a matter of paths chosen...or paths found. A comparative example of positive versus negative paths I like to use when talking with parents is that of children who later become Olympic level swimmers.

Ask yourself, what child gets up at 4 a.m. every morning to get to the pool by 5 a.m. so they can partake in swimming training before attending school? Indeed, this does sound a tad like an addiction.

In fact, it is. But, it is a rather healthy application, I would say: one with purpose, direction, and potential for extremely positive reward. Bottom line, a component of the addiction signature in children and adolescence is merely the "H" in ADHD *and it does not need to be negative.* If such "excess" of kinetic energy and need for external stimulation can be properly directed, it can, and often does, lead to the greatest of achievements (see multiple works of Hartmann).[87] [88]

If such "excess" of kinetic energy and need for external stimulation can be properly directed, it can, and often does, lead to the greatest of achievements.

Direction Versus Correction

Another discussion I often have with parents is the relative weight of direction versus correction of a child's hyperactivity or inattentiveness to what they perceive as the mundane. We often discuss medications such as stimulants and whose objectives are we filling by effectively sedating a child for attention inabilities in the classroom. What has been forgotten in the modern, or pharmaceutical era, is that "hyperactivity" is merely the sign of a busy brain that is significantly more inquisitive and often demands higher than average stimulation.

Yes, we need to help children train their abilities to sustain the mundane. Most of modern life, if we really think about it, is rather mundane: learning our times tables, doing our grooming and chores, finishing what we start, driving within the speed limit... Indeed we need to learn how to do these things, how to focus on them; otherwise we will not be productive people as children or later as adults. But that does not mean we all have to become choirboys, hands folded on our laps in angelic attention or production. We *DO NOT* want to train out the healthy pursuit of novelty or excitement.

In my treatment modality of therapeutic intervention (neurotherapy), we have found if the hyperactive signature is reduced slightly *and* the child is provided with appropriate opportunity for stimulation, the hyperactivity becomes significantly less problematic. I am happy to say we have many successful direction stories, of previously "problematic hyperactive" children who go on to win whacky science competitions, or become elite athletes and entrepreneurs. Note, no delusions here. Due to their inquisitive nature, these kids are still extremely difficult (AKA very time and energy consuming) to parent and to educate. They will, and do, require higher than average parental and educator attention. But they are worth it!

Back to Alpha

What my current clinical data is showing is that Alpha brainwave plasticity bears quite a resemblance to Theta/Beta brainwave fragility. What is currently happening with "artistic" Alpha and i-tech appears to be is very similar to what happens to "hyperactive" Theta/Beta brainwaves and the potential for addiction. Just as a busy brain signature can be hijacked by positive addiction (such as sports) or negative addiction (such as street drugs or alcohol), robust Alpha brainwave response can bloom in creativity or be hijacked by i-tech.

A Game of Semantics

Apart from the lexicon or word itself, the only fundamental difference between drive and addiction is outcome. The underlying behavior and brain wiring is identical. Addiction is the relentless pursuit of something negative (*behavior or substance that is pursued with disregard for its potential to harm*), while drive is the relentless pursuit of something perceived as positive. There are even crossover categories such as workaholic. Positive? Negative? It all depends on who is judging the relative value of outcome: the individual, their spouse, an MD, the community, the bank?

Similarly, Alpha can explode in creative process (music, art, dance, woodworking, robotics, higher levels of mathematics, the sciences, or architecture) or be directed to digital media. An aptitude for creative or innovative processing is the hook. Identical to addiction, it is a matter of what "fish" the hook first catches while trolling in the water.

In adolescence, both street drugs and sport will quiet the hyperactive brain ... it is merely a question of which one is most accessible and hence which one the child finds first.

In adolescence, both street drugs and sport will quiet the hyperactive brain by feeding it the stimulation it is seeking. For most, it is merely a question of which one is most accessible and hence which one the child finds first. In essence it is about positive versus negative opportunity, in critical periods of childhood and adolescence.

The Gaming Connection

The gaming industry knows of the connection of gaming to (innovative) processing and efficient Alpha brainwaves. As such, gaming is often touted as positive, improving reaction time and working memory. One study, for example, found that individuals with very efficient Alpha, peak frequency of 10Hz (*which in my field we know is otherwise associated with superior intelligence and innovative thinking*), were found to learn gaming at a significantly faster rate; reaction time and working memory further became superior with gaming.[89] They are correct, but I believe we must be very, very, cautious when interpreting and applying the implications of research findings to larger learning platforms.

From my clinical perspective, I would say that efficient brains are significantly more efficient at learning, including the learning of gaming. Period! I have no doubt of the veracity of the data that says this also improves processing speed, but to what end?

For those of us working in the trenches with children and families battling learning disabilities and behavioral challenges, the critical question of how these "improvements" affect us outside of gaming is still largely unanswered by the industry. My query is not satisfied by proof provided by standardized tests that measure spatial planning or processing speed (presumably of individuals without challenges). I want to know *how* this practically externalizes in real life. In my clinical work I am seeing that there is a critical trade-off in innovative or creative process, attention spans, and socialization. And this aspect is not being addressed by the industry.

A couple of studies question precisely this: the tangible transference of skills and the cause-effect connection of gaming to higher cognitive and sensorimotor skills. Boot, Blakely, and Simons reevaluated a series of studies routinely referenced in public media proclaiming external benefits of gaming. They found that systematically the studies were methodologically flawed. Indeed the studies found that many gamers had superior perceptual and cognitive abilities but there was no evidence whatsoever that these abilities were due to gaming nor that they transferred to skills other than gaming. When they tried to reproduce the work (without methodological flaws), they found they could not. Much as I have found in my clinical research, their only solid finding is that such brains are apparently disproportionately attracted to gaming. Boot, Blakely, and Simons conclude that until further evidence proves otherwise, the only benefit of gaming it is that it is fun.[90]

The debate is not over, not by far. It appears we, the psychologists, researchers, and game promoters, will staunchly defend our relative positions, often finding and thereafter arguing the exact same data points as positive versus negative. It is a matter of position and perspective, and, yes, vested interest. Case in point, yet another study has found routine first shooter game players (e.g., Call of Duty and Assassin's Creed) to be superior in the learning of sensorimotor skills: the learning of complex patterns.[91] However, what the authors and subsequent media feeds proclaim as positive, I in turn see as potentially negative, or at the very least rather neutral in day-to-day life. Again it is a matter of perspective. Here, I play my broken record, asking everyone to read the small print of research and ponder the gross implications of "findings."

In this study gamers were found equal to non-gamers in the learning of new or unfamiliar sensorimotor tasks. Gamers, however, were significantly better at learning and thereafter following repetitive motions. When patterns changed again, back to unlearned or new patterns, there was once again no difference in the abilities of gamers and non-gamers.

The conclusions drawn, however, were most positive. The superior abilities of first person shooter gamers to learn repetitive motion or repetitive patterns were touted as key skills for the most prestigious of professions, none other than laparoscopic surgeons or those conducting remote surgeries.

I don't know about you, but my thinking varies. Yes, I would want my surgeon to be masterful at learned routine, particularly when using equipment requiring high precision manual control, but I would equally want him or her to be able to spontaneously act or react to the unforeseen, say when a surgery is not quite on target or when patterns unexpectedly go off course. Again, to me at least, repetitive tasking skills seem more appropriate to factory line workers than surgeons. Another analogy would be to driving. If I were a Formula One driver, indeed this is not only a necessary skill but a critical one. Knowing the various circuits in each participating city by rote is a skill central to not only surviving, but to excelling, to winning. But were I in a car, on a supremely winding road, I would want superior spontaneous or reactive skills, not rote ones, whether the road was known to me or not.

The larger question is not how many of us become Formula One drivers versus factory workers, or even laparoscopic or remote surgeons, but how many of us become drivers of our own cars or passengers in others where rote and reactive skills are both implicated. Which skills do we want weighing heavier in the big picture?

In this context, I also can't resist an irony-laden poke. Do you really want the person potentially responsible for saving your life, in laparoscopic or remote surgery, to have acquired their skills at precision movement in games that rewarded them for efficiently learning how to kill? I would prefer such skills were learned a little more traditionally, or at the very least in virtual environments that save not destroy. Here my sarcasm is not veiled.

Similarly, veiling the absurdity of the analogy of surgery to search and destroy games with counter-arguments of team building, the learning of cooperative skills, and the like, fuels the exasperation of those of us trying to help children and educate parents. For any professional with a grain of social intelligence or empathic reasoning, this type of extension of research results is not only laughable, but downright insulting. Yet this is exactly what we are being told; no wonder parents can't make sense of it all.

Tying back to the role of Alpha, and the learning, and thereafter application, of creative versus routine processing: my clinical work clearly implicates that the learning of rote, or the exclusive training of the brain for rote, at some point supersedes creative process. We learn to follow (only) the path of the program and have decreased abilities to act reactively, spontaneously, or with independent thought. Arguably, we become programmed. Advancements in science (including medicine and surgical procedures) originate from the rational integration of learned information (e.g., schooling and experience) with new or presenting information and resulting thoughts such as: "What if we try this? Would it be more efficient, more successful, more helpful?" This is a mental (creative-cognitive) process far beyond rote, and more importantly, one that can be blocked by rote thinking, and routine rote (or programmed) processing.

The Narrowing of Minds

How do you measure creativity if you never find it in the first place? As mentioned earlier, a concerning gaming glitch I have noticed over the past five to eight years is that youth are progressively less aware of their creative potential. Today, many kids don't lose the creativity, they never find it!

They never become aware of the talent they potentially possess. Instead the "talent" is applied to gaming (and all i-media for that matter). This to me is a great tragedy: not only to the individual but to society as a whole. We potentially are losing our greatest innovative thinkers. This form of intelligence should be applied to science and art AKA invention, not to the following of a computer program, AKA computer games.

Now before I sound like an old fart, I have absolutely nothing against fun, including mindless fun with no learning objectives and no potential for anything except the participant's enjoyment (and that includes gaming). It all has its place. In fact we don't play enough anymore. But that is another chapter. My issue with computer or digital gaming, including educational gaming, is what I refer to as the double-edged delusion: first, that the games and all i-tech are helping us learn exquisite skills; and second, that excessive usage does us no harm.

Learning and Creative Space in Educational Gaming

So beyond the great debate of improved or not improved sensorimotor skills, how do i-games and computer programs change thinking, creative and otherwise?

A clear example of thwarted creativity can be seen in the classic educational game of groupings. In grouping games, a child is shown a few elements, and must decide from other elements how to complete the set. Take for example, three yellow squares, followed by the choice between a pink square and a banana. According to the program, the pink square is the "correct" answer as it is the identical geometric shape. The banana is the "incorrect" answer; it is the wrong shape. But what if the child was thinking color, not shape, never mind some other factor?

A child who chooses the banana is told by the program that he or she is incorrect. The child is further not asked to explain why the banana would fit the set (no opportunity to rationalize or explain alternate logic).

But it does not end here. The child is also penalized for exploratory or potentially innovative thinking. This reward-penalization polarization is my greatest concern. If this process is repeated often enough, the child will essentially reprogram his or her processing to think as the program does, pruning human thinking to a specific form of computer thinking (e.g., unilinear instead of multifactorial). This is basic conditioning, psychology 101, and rather frightening to be doing to little brains in the name of learning.

If this process is repeated often enough, the child will essentially reprogram his or her processing to think as the program does, pruning human thinking to a specific form of computer thinking (e.g., unilinear instead of multifactorial).

Changing Educational Orientation

With these types of educational games, children also become oriented toward scoring rather than learning. It quickly becomes more of a gambling game than a learning game (with 50/50 odds of winning or losing). And that, also, changes the brain's orientation. In essence the learning orientation changes from inquiry and exploration of possibilities that may be proven true, possible, or untrue (true scientific enquiry) to polarized right/wrong, pass/fail, score/don't score. It is the difference between fostering an inquisitive, scientific mind versus a regurgitating mind that only repeats what has been programmed: a mind and hence a person that does not think, question, or explore on their own. But they are entertained – very, very entertained.

When left creative space, kids will come up with the most interesting logic, if we allow them said space to do so. To uninhibited or unbound young minds, possibilities are endless, and you want your children to go there as that is where true intelligence is fostered; e.g., "they were banana flavored candies, and the pink mint did not taste the same." That is the budding mind of a future chef, a perfumer, a sommelier, designer, or a product marketing expert rather than a factory line worker, rubber stamper, or a paper pusher.

What to Do?

Water the Seed!

When left to the "correct/incorrect" or any polarized classifications of a program, a child is explicitly limited by the format or intention of the program. Such limitations stifle innovative, never mind creative, thinking. The solution I believe is simple: if you do choose to use educational games, play them with your child. This will allow your child voice beyond that of the program(mer). In my experience, it is the human interaction that provides the greater part of the learning.

Catch: Ensure that you are actually playing with your child, truly interacting, not merely engaging with a device and your child just happens to be there doing the same. Also please ensure that you are not being exclusively directed by the program and its imposed limitations and...well, program, for example, that you do not merely vocalize or reinforce what the program dictates (e.g., ask "why the banana?" not merely state "no, the correct choice is the pink square").

Unfortunately a few studies on reading programs or reading games have found the latter, that parents do not explore with their children, but indeed merely reinforce the program. Further, that interactive e-reading of children's books or reading programs completely changed the orientation as well as the interpersonal interaction of parents to children.

Dr. Parish-Morris and her team[92] found that when e-reading, parents did not dialogue read, meaning they did not focus on the story or discuss its content or any ideas it brought up. They interacted with the device and only the device. The device and the program ruled. Parents would further physically restrain children, stopping them from pushing buttons that were not in the correct order, directing their children how to use the program, how to use the device, not to absorb or follow the story. This is precisely the integration versus interference argument explored in Chapter Two. In this specific case, "reading" became rule, program, or game following directed or mitigated by a parent. This does not sound much like learning to read or positive emotional bonding (snuggly reading time) to me...

I don't know about you, but at that point if I had a completely free hour to play with a child, I would prefer to race toy cars, dance around pretending to be the King and Queen of Sheba, snuggle up reading a paper book, draw fireflies, have a tickling war, bake cookies, or get outside. Kids have enough structure already in school; unstructured play at home provides endless possibilities for learning, never mind the solidifying of attachment and other positive emotional bonds.

If you need any extra convincing, I find this quote from Maria, a thirty-year-old participant in my study on i-addiction, most powerful. It expresses firsthand the experience of frustration and sadness due to the loss of creativity.

> When I was in my teens and very early 20s my creativity level was very high. This has declined drastically and caused me a tremendous amount of anxiety and deep depression. It recently dawned on me that there seems to be a direct correlation to the amount of time I spend online and the drop in my creativity and imaginative abilities. It became harder and harder to get that electric sensation in my body that comes from creative thinking, and at this point in time it feels almost impossible. I have tried to cut off exposure to any media devices in an attempt to regain this ability but those attempts have failed.

And now back to Alpha.

Omnipotent Alpha

The role of Alpha brainwaves is by no means limited to creativity and innovative processing. Alpha is a most unique and powerful frequency in all that it governs. One of its unique features is its role in what we refer to as attentive idling. Accordingly, it is often the frequency we train for in elite military pilots, top executives, and professional athletes. In essence, Alpha is the Peak Performance brainwave, and many Olympic athletes and elite teams in sports have publicly announced their use of the modality toward their success(es).

One of the key features of Alpha brainwave efficiency is readiness: the ability to be perfectly at rest yet be able to jump to action instantly when required. For a pilot, hypervigilance causes fatigue and hence inefficiency, leading to higher potential for critical error. A fighter pilot must be at rest, performing his or her flight duties in calm but able to switch on instantly when (sometimes literally) under fire. Same for elite athletes: they must be at (brain) rest, observant, and in position or in the mindset to act instantly when the ball (or opportunity to strike/perform) is theirs. When Alpha is efficient, we do not tire so quickly (or miss our mark) as the brain is efficiently transitioning from rest to action, rest to action. In my clinical experience, this is also a critical component in executive burnout. Those with the "addiction signature" – AKA drive and efficient Alpha – don't tend to burn out so quickly. Those with the drive signature and inefficient Alpha do!

Apart from Alpha brainwave efficiency (*or speed of Alpha recovery*), the role of Alpha also changes distinctly depending on brain location and the relative strength of the wave (*location, amplitude, and ratios*). Increasingly I am seeing that excessive usage of digital media also recruits Alpha brainwaves elsewhere in the brain: in brain regions where *we don't want more*, brain regions where robust Alpha does exactly the opposite of what we want. Enter High Frontal Alpha ADHD.

What is Efficiency?

In my study on i-addiction, just as the participants had voraciously strong creativity and innovation signatures (*high amplitude Alpha brainwaves in the right place under the right condition*), they also had uniformly strong Alpha brainwaves in the wrong place, under the wrong condition (*high relative amplitudes frontally*). This is the brainwave signature for High Frontal Alpha ADHD, and 89% of the participants had it!

High Frontal Alpha ADHD has the attributes of inattention, poor organization and planning, daydreaming, and excessive mind chatter. Perhaps also of interest, we see relatively similar symptoms in a variant of this (*elevated Low/High Alpha brainwave ratios @ location Fz*), another EEG marker found in ADHD, but also common to those with age-related cognitive decline (dementia) and uniformly seen in marijuana smokers. Prior to gaming and i-media, we typically saw both of these forms of ADHD undiagnosed in females: fitting gender bias under the negative cultural stereotype of ditzy girls, as opposed to being recognized as an attention deficit as in the case of their male counterparts.[93]

What We Want and Where We Want It

All this points to why I am most concerned regarding the gaming industry's research that gaming promotes (positive) changes in Alpha brainwaves. If it is only augmentation of peak frequency 10Hz Alpha (*associated with brain efficiency and by proxy intelligence*), the robustness of the Alpha response (*AKA the creative/innovative signature*), and the recovery speed (*moving from idle to action at impeccable speed*), it is most positive – but, if, and only if, it does not hijack the creative application(s), and surely if it also does not make us disorganized, spacey, or with hopelessly busy brains when not engaged.

My preliminary research findings unfortunately indicate that gaming and all excessive applications of digital media are not complementary; in clinical populations, they both supplant creative process *and* decrease the ability to sustain focus by increasing frontal Alpha brainwaves. They decrease innovation and decrease focus on that which is not overtly stimulating.

The gaming industry does us quite a disservice by touting the positive features of gaming in individuals with already efficient brains or those who game professionally as testers for the industry. I also find that research showing that the average brain functions, or reacts, to gaming differently than that of a professional gamer (or tester for the industry) is largely ignored.

Aptitudes and Addictions

An example I like to use again is that of alcohol. Research has found that different areas of the brain light up with alcohol consumption, based on our relationship with alcohol. For the alcoholic, predictably, reward centers and pathways associated with addiction light up; for the sommelier, cognitive and some emotional centers light up. For the naïve consumer, AKA most of us who enjoy a drink socially, the emotional centers light up.[94] The same is true of gaming. Professional gamers and game testers use cognitive processing while gaming. For addicted gamers, or those at risk of excessive usage, the areas of the brain regulating impulse tend to override those regulating reason. The addiction centers light up.

Scientific Corner: Research Findings

Limited research specifically examines brain function and IA. fMRI studies to date focus on Internet gaming and have found that IA in gaming shares many of the same neurobiological mechanisms as substance abuse and pathological gambling. Dopaminergic pathways are implicated (Weinstein, 2010)[95] as are multiple systems and regions associated with reward circuitry.

Regions of the brain activated with online gaming addiction appear to overlap with those activated with cue-induced craving in substance dependence. Cue-induced gaming urges share the same neural substrates, including the right orbitofrontal cortex, right nucleus accumbens, bilateral anterior cingulate, medial frontal cortex, right dorsolateral prefrontal cortex, and right caudate nucleus (Ko, Lui, et al., 2009)[96]. Han et al. (2011)[97] also found cue-induced activation of the dorsolateral prefrontal, orbitofrontal cortex, parahippocampal gyrus, and the thalamus. This circuitry is also activated in pathological gambling as well as substance abuse (Kalivas and Volkow, 2005[98]).

Zhou et al. (2009)[99] examined morphological changes in gray matter density in adolescents diagnosed with IA. They found lower density in the left anterior cingulated cortex, the left posterior cingulated cortex, the left lingual gyrus, and the left insula areas associated with the modulation of emotional behavior. Insula dysfunction is also highly implicated in urge control (risk, rewards, and motivation) as related to addiction. Liu et al. (2010[100]) found increased regional homogeneity in individuals with IA including enhanced synchronization among the cerebellum, brainstem, limbic and frontal lobes, and apical lobe associated with reward pathways. Lui et al. (2010) also found increased homogeneity and enhanced synchronization in encephalic regions, cerebellum, brainstem, limbic lobe, and apical lobe, which they also related to reward pathways.

Han, Kim, Lee, Min, and Renshaw (2010)[101] found increased activity in the prefrontal cortex. During cue exposure in gaming, they found increased activity in orbitofrontal cortex and anterior cingulated cortex, the same regions affected in substance abuse. They conclude that excessive gaming changes brain activity much in the same way as substance abuse. In a study examining variation in brain volume in professional gamers versus game addicts, Han, Lyoo, and Renshaw (2012)[102] found higher volume in left thalamic gray matter, and decreased gray matter in the inferior temporal gyri, left inferior gyrus, and right middle occipital gyrus. They conclude that volume lateralized to the left is associated with gaming addiction whereas decreased gray matter in the occipital cortex and inferior temporal cortex were common to all players. Han et al. further suggest that playing styles (impulsive vs. calculated play) of individuals who play games professionally versus individuals with gaming addiction are responsible for left to right variation. Both forms of extensive gaming, however, do appear to affect brain development, specifically the maturation of the visual cortex.

Ruobing, Xianming, and Xiapeng (2008)[103] differentiated between the activation of brain regions associated with the processing and integration of information and those associated with addiction. Both types of activation were elevated in adolescents with gaming IA. All affected regions were again associated with reward systems. Dong, De Vito, Huang, and Du (2012)[104] found higher volume in the left posterior cingulate cortex and the bilateral thalamus.

In sum, brain imaging studies on IA gaming have collectively found that as with other addictions, multiple systems and regions involved in reward and executive function are implicated.

The Good News

The good news is the brain is plastic. We can modify the Alpha brainwave deregulation rather quickly if we catch it fast enough and parents realize the potential if not actual severity of the problem. The catch is most parents don't. I am happy (indirectly, I should qualify) that I now see children, youth, and adolescents brought in specifically for i-addiction, most often gaming, texting, and searching. I am very troubled however by parents' complacency.

Many parents are prepared to pay for treatment for their child to "get better," but they are not prepared to take parental action to ensure its success. Translation: many parents want or expect their children to auto-regulate but they will not remove the devices from the family home or their personal possession, nor will they monitor. I have only bad news here. If parents don't take very severe action, the child will not disengage from i-tech. Period.

Forget analogies of ice cream to broccoli and how children don't auto-regulate when provided such a choice. I've been known to use some pretty severe analogies to other addictive substances to get the message across. We are talking about addiction, a new form of addiction commandeering not only teens but little children.

So I say, think cocaine, heroin, or alcohol. Think you are leaving a bottle of vodka on the table and asking an alcoholic not to drink it, and who bought the vodka in the first place? Bottom line, parents must be prepared to either remove devices from their children's reach or monitor them severely, *and* not purchase any more, or otherwise allow other friends or family to gift said items to their children. If the devices are left available, point blank, any intervention, neurotherapy or otherwise, will not work. There will be brief improvements and then the brain will deregulate once again; educational deficits and behavioral challenges will reappear.

This note from a parent tells all:

> *Hi*
>
> *Happy New Year!*
>
> *I am writing about [Brian]. I am concerned, because recently we are seeing him exhibit some of his past behaviors. His OCD [Obsessive Compulsive Disorder] is coming back and he is having frustration outbursts.*
>
> *At Christmas we got a Wii U video game and initially allowed him to play it only on the weekends. We were cautious and timed it. Then we relaxed the rules and let him play more often. I fear this is making his OCD come back. He is not compulsively washing his hands again but has a lot of the other symptoms. He is becoming frustrated a lot quicker and has had a few outbursts at school.*
>
> *I am going to completely remove the video games again so he can try to get back to a more relaxed state, but I am not sure if this will be enough. I don't want his behavior to get worse. Should I bring him back for more treatment?*
>
> *I know his reaction to taking away the game is going to be horrible and hard. He will obsess about me letting him play. He will always bring it up and beg for only a few minutes.*
>
> *I don't know if this is the right thing to do, but I know that getting the game is the only thing that has changed in his life.*

This email was received toward the end of February, indicating that merely two months' exposure to gaming was responsible for the return of the symptoms for which this family originally sought treatment. Note that the game was on Wii, not Halo or Grand Theft Auto or any of the other violent or otherwise aggressive games commonly attributed to emotional deregulation.

What to Do?

For gaming addiction, I recommend cold turkey followed by permanent abstinence: identical to what is typically recommended for any other "non-essential" addictive substance or behavior. For other i-media, it is a little more difficult as the technologies are fully integrated in modern life. The most apt example unfortunately is that of children and adolescents who have developed eating disorders. You can't tell the bulimic adolescent or the morbidly obese child to stop eating; they must learn to regulate the ingestive behavior with the aid of severe and systematic regulation from parents where they routinely fail. For the bulimic, this would mean monitoring for vomiting post ingestion and not buying (or providing access to a plethora of) ice cream, cake, cookies, chips, cereal, or whatever the individual can and does binge on in the home. Parenting for children and adolescents with eating disorders requires choice restriction, portion control, *and* monetary restriction. With i-tech, it means restricting all usage that is not scholastically imperative. And, as with food to money, so is gaming to friends. Meaning, just as a parent would need to watch that morbidly obese Johnny does not just go to Auntie Jane's and eat twenty cookies, or to the corner store with his allowance and buy eight chocolate bars, they need to control that i-tech Johnny does not go to Amir's house for the afternoon and play four hours on his game of choice.

Now, all that said, for those parents who catch the problem early and are prepared to take parental action, I have nothing but good news. But again, no delusions here...it ain't easy...Addiction never is.

Meet Cassandra

Cassandra was a lost young woman of twenty, the eldest of three siblings all brought in for treatment. Cassandra was still living at home. She was not attending school, nor was she working. She spent most of her days sleeping and moping around the house, and was not contributing in any manner whatsoever to the household. She complained of chronic headaches, insomnia, and erratic eating habits, and was concerned about her weight. She was feeling depressed, restless, and anxious. Cassandra had further classified herself as a perfectionist as well as artistic on her intake forms.

Cassandra's EEG brainmap matched her descriptive profile. She had the signature for troubles with self-quieting, insomnia, and predisposition to addiction (*a low Theta/Beta brainwave ratio in the occiput*), depression (*over 15% disparity in brainwave amplitudes across the frontal lobes*), and perseveration (*a HiBeta/Beta brainwave ratio frontally*). She also had a magnificent increase in Alpha waves with her eyes closed: the artist signature. What Cassandra's EEG also showed was deregulated Alpha frontally.

All the bells went off. Cassandra had my two telltale signs of excessive use of digital media (*robust Alpha brainwave response and deregulated Alpha frontally*). Cassandra also had the full EEG cluster pattern I had found in my study of self-confessed i-addicts (*addiction signature, depression signature, high-frontal ADHD signature, and perseveration/obsessive signature*).

I took a risk alienating this young woman with potentially antagonistic directness. I looked her straight in the eyes and asked about her online usage, and then said, "Stop it"! I knew I had hit the bulls-eye by parental reaction. I followed up with explaining that excessive i-usage was exacerbating if not causing all her problems; she needed to get offline and reengage with the outside world. She needed to get a job or go back to school, period! I also told her parents that the not so minor educational issues of their two younger boys paled in comparison; Cassandra was their greatest concern. She was at extreme risk of failure to launch.

I am happy to report that within five sessions (five weeks) Cassandra had changed dramatically, as had her brainwaves. Alpha became totally regulated, reducing by 173.8%. I must also give credit where credit is due. Cassandra's parents took the information seriously, and parented seriously. They clearly recognized the difference between parental support and empathy for transitioning from high school to the next stage of life versus enabling stagnation. They firmly recognized that Cassandra was at risk of developing severe pathology in the form of depression. As a result Cassandra jumped to the plate. She sought out educational options and applied for jobs. Cassandra is now faced with the wonderful decision between learning the entry level rules of the working world and continuing her education. The cluster pattern responsible for her other symptoms can now be addressed, and I trust successfully, through further therapy.

Cassandra was an easy client; she was from an engaged and loving family that was not looking for a magic bullet. Perhaps most importantly, once the antagonist was recognized, both parents and child alike took responsibility for their part in the development and maintenance of the problem and acted on it. They did not bow to anxiety or depression as an excuse for inaction, and acknowledged the excessive use of i-tech for what it was. Cassandra was also "easy" because the problem had not yet invaded to a critical degree. She had only been bingeing online since graduating from high school: a year at best.

The True Battle

The catch is that many children and youth have been involved in excessive consumption of i-media, gaming, etc., since early childhood. For these individuals, disengaging is quite a different challenge. They have no other hobbies, limited or atypical socialization skills, and no friends other than those online or in the gaming community (on- or offline). These children and youth are very seriously deregulated, and will go through significant withdrawal. If your brain has been trained for and has not developed other orientation, nothing, and I mean nothing, stimulates to the degree of gaming and i-tech. They will be bored out of their skulls, restless, angry, and have no concept whatsoever of how to self-entertain or engage in other activities.

For these children cold turkey is the only resolution. I not so subtly suggest parents have i-tech devices "break" rather than discuss and rationalize with their children how and why the devices are not good and why they will be removing them. It's a softer presentation and easier for parents to manage behaviorally than explicitly taking the gaming devices or other i-tech away. For one, "addicts," children or not, tend not to be particularly rational in the face of their addiction. Two, figuratively speaking, little children often just want ice cream or candy and they will tantrum, beg, and scream to wear parents down, relentlessly so. They could not care less about nutritional value or obesity. Same with i-tech and ADHD, emotional regulation, social skills or whatever reason a parent is seeking therapy for their child; in the face of gaming loss, these are completely irrelevant to them. Bottom line, the little white lie is easier for parents to implement.

Every once in a while, however, parents choose the "rational" route, including asking me, "the knowledgeable doctor," to support them in explaining to their child why he or she will no longer be permitted to game. I know what is coming, but parents in this situation have no clue. It is disastrous!

Once, in this precise scenario, a not so little boy, let's call him Ali, started screaming at me in full voice crying, blustering, "I hate you!"; "you are ruining my life!" There was a little not so nice name-calling too. From the waiting room one would think I was murdering the child. Ali's mother's initial response was shame regarding his behavior toward me and, accordingly, she started to parent her son vis-à-vis how he was addressing me. She was missing the point. This outburst was not the concern, not by far.

Ali then proceeded to moan, curl up in fetal position, and roll on the floor in full tears as if in physical pain, crying "what am I going to do"; "I have nothing to do." When his mother went to comfort him he started to get physical. He hit his mother and then proceeded to twist the blinds on my office door. The positive, I suppose, is that with this reaction, Ali's mother finally realized the severity of the situation. This emotional and physical reaction was indeed what one would expect with gaming addiction. I am happy to say that within two weeks Ali turned. He happily bopped into my office two weeks later telling of all the new things he was doing as well as doing better in school.

Now I do not want to leave you with this Pollyanna image; there are many others who do not, or at least take considerably longer (months in fact) to emotionally disengage from not only the perceived loss, but also the actual loss, of gaming. The part also not mentioned is Ali's mother had one solid week of absolute hell on her hands before her son calmed. What was witnessed in my office was only the beginning.

Please note that excessive i-tech utilization has the potential to negatively affect any and all children and youth: those already battling serious mental health issues such as Brian and his Obsessive Compulsive Disorder; otherwise typical children such as Franco and Ali with some mild attentional difficulties; as well as Cassandra in a rather typical phase of post-adolescent transition. But, over time, most can and do re-adapt to healthy and integrated use of i-tech for schooling and pleasure.

When to Say, No, No, Never!

Now, there is one absolute exception. Any child who is on the Autistic or Asperger's spectrum is at disproportionate risk for total derailment with any and all use of i-tech. At the clinic we routinely see completely thwarted socio-emotional and behavioral development not only due to the liabilities inherent to the disorders, but due to hyper-focus on digital devices to the exclusion of all other functional relationships.

If you have a child or a child with Autism or Asperger's under your care (parents, caretakers, teachers, grandparents, etc.), under no circumstances permit the child to engage with i-tech, any i-tech. Although most tempting, as indeed such children are very time and attention demanding and NOTHING else grabs their attention as does i-tech, please note over time it will invariably make your job (parenting, caretaking, and educating) dramatically more intensive. It will exacerbate all symptoms and severely compromise further socio-emotional development. I cannot make this point more strongly![105]

A counter-argument I often hear, and wish to address directly, is that children on either spectrum will need i-tech to integrate socially, even more than children who are not. The argument is based upon the premise that children on the spectrum(s) are indeed socially and emotionally compromised and i-tech will facilitate socialization, learning, and integration in society. i-tech is seen as the facilitator as opposed to the thwarter. What i-tech actually does, however, is support and exacerbate brain miswiring as opposed to link it. Individuals can surely learn how to functionally use technologies for work and communication as needed when older, when the brain is more fully developed and when they, and those supporting them, can objectively select which aspects help versus harm.

And Now the Truly Dark Side...

There is a second side to this, perhaps this time a little more overtly pernicious in the development of addiction, anxiety, and lack of focus. The Internet, and modern technology in general, supports gaming that is formatted, or intentionally designed, to overtly or covertly penalize disengagement, and it is a little stronger than needing or wanting to finish a game level.

In many games, players can lose territory or property they won or bought, let down team members, and lose social connections when they disengage or do not show up for play. Some games will have zombies attack and tear down your constructions if you are offline too long. Teams or leagues will lose without the "special power" of a missing player. Others will not keep scores or record level of achievement unless a process is completed before disengaging. Hence the cries of "but I have to," "all my friends are there," or "just another minute," or ten, or twenty and even the anger when asked, or required to stop. We must recognize that the child or adolescent (any gamer) is actually losing something by disengaging. Under these conditions games stop being just fun: there are duties that come with play.

Traditional games played online without monetary exchange (e.g., bridge, solitaire) may still be an attractive and at-risk activity due to limitless availability and accessibility. However, unlike many online social fantasy and team-based search-and-destroy games (other than a void of how to occupy oneself), there is no perceived investment loss, social loss, or scoring penalization when an individual withdraws or stays away from play. In contrast, the very structure of many online games, much like in traditional gambling, reinforces addiction.[106]

> ...the very structure of many online games, much like in traditional gambling, reinforces addiction.

When my clients come in enthusiastically talking of a fantastic game they can play and enjoy for a couple of hours a week, just like a board game, or tennis, tag, guitar, Lego, or anything that for that matter does not overtly penalize disengagement, commandeer recess, or trigger the anxiety or the addiction button, I will change my professional stance. In the meantime, I conservatively suggest that, knowing the potential pitfalls, one really restrict usage, and perhaps subsequently enjoy them less. A good measure would be to not engage in any i-activity that leaves you or your child empty, socially isolated, bored, or agitated without it.

For little children, professional voices are rather unanimous: *NO* i-media or screens whatsoever before the age of *two*. For most this is now *four*. Many of us, including myself, have conservatively augmented this to *six* because, as will be presented in the following chapters, the potential developmental perils are too high. For older children and adults, the healthy cut-off point appears to be one hour per day. More than this appears connected with increased anxiety, agitation, general restlessness, and related boredom when not "connected."

For older children and adults, the healthy cut-off point appears to be one hour per day. More than this appears connected with increased anxiety, agitation, general restlessness, and related boredom when not "connected."

CHAPTER SEVEN

The Good, the Bad, and the Neutral

And now, it is time to explore medium and method, delivery and processing systems. Many parents and educators do see a benefit to educational television and now gaming, and rightly so. In the realm of television, shows produced by National Geographic and child favorites such as *Sesame Street* and *How Things are Made* are touted for their educational benefits; so too are games.

I have already addressed some of the pitfalls of educational games such as polarized or uni-linear learning that can thwart creativity and innovative process. In this chapter and those following I will build an argument for the importance of people: that i-tech should not replace human interaction or human process; that if we choose technology, it should be in addition to, not a replacement for, educators or parents. For those supporting media and i-tech as a positive addition to family life, parental involvement is still key. Kids don't only watch and learn the good stuff.

Much like a host and its parasite, some pretty negative stuff is lurking online and on TV too. Parental participation, including active gaming and viewing with children, mitigates against potentially negative social and developmental effects.[107] It also ensures that we stay present, bonded, together.

Pro Viewing and Pro Gaming

In terms of gaming, for many years James Gee[108] was often cited in argument critiquing the anti-gaming position. He believes gaming receives a lot of bad press due to violent games when in fact many games are pro-social and educational. In support of his, and other respected professional opinions, there are now many studies that concur with this thesis. There is even a new study out that states violent gaming can induce not only improvements in sensorimotor skills (as presented earlier) but pro-social behavior by producing guilt.[109]

In the realm of education, Gee believes gaming can be a more effective tool of teaching than standard schooling as games allow for great exploration and deep learning through experimental and contextual learning. He points out that many games are collaborative, teaching collective problem solving and teamwork. As one is learning with others, it also teaches about emotional ranges of behavior. However, as Gee himself notes, in order for this form of learning to be effective, and a positive learning model, children still need mentors. Children need to debrief, and discuss the learning process, the views, and feelings of other individuals. Even what Gee refers to as good games do not provide this out of the box. Something or someone has to encourage reflection.

I have no argument with what Gee and others profess per se, except I do not see this happening. The vast majority of parents are not engaging with their children with these games, and, as such, the argument becomes moot. When engaging by themselves or with peers only, children do not tend to reflect, they merely absorb. Unfortunately, a parental (and educator) abdication often occurs with media and i-tech. Children typically watch TV and game as parents do other work, chores, or engage on their own i-devices. In classrooms, I see the applications being applied as a substitute or replacement for, not in addition to, educator attention.

Gee and others also speak to the entertainment value of educational gaming. Children enjoy gaming, and the medium can engage them for longer periods of time. This argument is often used as the proof of the educational value or positive value of media in general. There is mounting evidence that being aroused (clapping or giggling along) or mesmerized (unrelenting attention) does not necessarily translate into being truly engaged or learning. Studies routinely show that information delivered by devices does not stick to the same degree as that being delivered by people. Nowhere is this more evident than in language learning in very young children. It appears there needs to be some sort of wiring between social function and linguistic function for language learning to succeed. Language through i-tech does not trigger the "social" wiring and hence neither the learning process.[110] [111]

It appears there needs to be some sort of wiring between social function and linguistic function for language learning to succeed.

Many, arguably Sigman,[112] argue vehemently against television executives (and game promoters) who promote children's programming as positive, entertaining, and educational. Sigman argues that a child's enjoyment should never be the basis upon which a parent or educator determines what is good for them. Enjoyment and attention are not synonymous with positive or innocuous. Children can also become engaged with and enjoy negative things.

Part of the role of parenting, caretaking, and education is to appropriately socialize children. Traditionally elders teach children what should inherently be bad/harmful, such as pulling a kitten's tail to see it jump and run (entertaining to the child and harmful to the animal) versus good/harmless, such as swinging a string to see the kitten jump and hide and jump again (entertaining to the child and entertaining to the animal). Media is consistently manipulating these boundaries. Like vaudeville theatre before it, a great part of the entertainment value of the medium is its ability to cross lines and play with the positive versus negative effect of behavior. This is exactly what early television and cartoons did. In traditional cartoons, Bugs Bunny punching Daffy Duck flat is most entertaining, and Daffy does not get hurt as he bounds back from his flattened state with gusto, and we laugh with gusto.

Changing Times

In traditional cartoons and programming, even in the absence of parental intervention, there were still numerous cues in the medium itself: the costuming, posturing, or voices told us so. Good cowboys wore white hats; bad cowboys wore black hats. I fear we have lost that now. Boundaries of character acceptability are becoming blurred with the exceptionally realistic quality of animation we see in gaming today. It is not a cartoon rabbit bashing a cartoon duck where they otherwise look, act, and talk funny; it's a near realistic animated guy bashing in the head of another realistic guy: blood, crack, and all.

Boundaries of character acceptability are becoming blurred with the exceptionally realistic quality of animation we see in gaming today.

In the absence of parental information to the contrary, realistic human figures in programming and gaming may be contributing to the desensitization and lack of understanding of consequences of potentially hurtful actions. Typically adults set up clear boundaries which children thereafter learn to follow. When children grow older and push the boundaries with peers in adolescence, they know precisely what boundaries they are experimenting with. Today, I question whether this still holds true.

There is a war going on out there regarding the negative, neutral, and even positive relationship between the playing of violent games and pro-social, anti-social, and overtly aggressive behavior. By now you can guess which side of the fence I stand on professionally, even more so now with such realistic gaming, or virtual reality.

Studies have proven that the more individuals identify with the character they are playing, the more desensitized they become. For example when females play violent games as a female, as opposed to male characters or avatars, the correlation with aggression is significantly higher[113] (which may loop into disinhibition). When the characters don't look like us or we don't project ourselves on them, we don't identify with them as much. Unfortunately the opposite also holds true.

What I am asking everyone to ponder is how we measure identification or self-projection: by gender, accent, looks, profession, ideology, our own fantasy, pseudo-reality, or self-projection as with self-built avatars? How do we know when someone will or will not identify, and is it worth the risk? The aforementioned study that found pro-social behavior with violent gaming in a US sample dealt with terrorist acts.[114] I am assuming, in current US culture at least, self-identification with terrorism, and terroristic acts, did not occur (hence the finding of guilt and pro-social behavior thereafter). But what about for those who do? What about those who do self-identify with violent behavior regardless of ideology?

Games as Therapy

I am further very concerned regarding explicit game development and marketing of games as not only beneficial but as therapeutic. Recently, I happened to see a Dutch interview of a North American doctor promoting a specific company's product and the generalized benefits of gaming for children, including their pro-social and pro-health benefits.[115] The jargon used was right on target including how games functioned in the "zone of proximal development" and how children broadened their analytic skills by "reappraising environments." The doctor even used the proper amount of scientific restraint including qualifiers: stating often that the industry too was still learning, studies contradicted each other, and we do not have all the information yet regarding the benefits or otherwise.

But her purpose was clear: she was promoting a game she and her cohorts had developed that was explicitly designed as a therapeutic tool to aid children in reducing anxiety. Now having just completed my chapter on anxiety, I thought this sounded quite interesting. Further, she was talking my language; her game involved brain entrainment, EEG work: Alpha to achieve states of calm and Beta for concentration.

As I continued to watch, I became quite concerned, then perturbed. First it appeared to me that the comprehensive role of Alpha in children was being grossly oversimplified. Alpha was being discussed as the relaxation wave (*without regard for location, amplitude, peak frequency, or band width parameters*). Remember there are some forms of Alpha you don't want a lot of (*increased Alpha is also associated with ADHD, poor planning and organization, and absent seizures, not only peak performance and relaxation*). Same with Beta; yes it is the focus wave, but it is also the anxiety wave, the hypervigilance wave, the "you can't quiet" wave. High frontal Beta is also highly correlated with perseveration, cognitive and emotive stubbornness or rigidity (*Obsessive Compulsive Disorders, Conduct Disorders and Autistic like symptoms*). Raising Beta can be a risky business.

In the interview, training brainwaves from the forehead, along with controlled breathing, was being portrayed as unilaterally positive, all one needed. Perhaps details were not relevant in a promotional interview. Perhaps she was simplifying, or being nonspecific, for a lay audience, and indeed was promoting refined Alpha/Beta training. Who knows, but it perpetrates the belief that it is simplistic, that potentially anyone can do "gaming therapy" at home, and that it is only positive – anything but!

But then there was a kicker (if one had the patience to watch the interview to its twenty-five-minute end, that is). When the doctor was asked if her children played games, she essentially said, "hell no." She allowed no screen time *whatsoever* during the week! She then recuperated, quite quickly explaining that she allowed gaming, three hours or so, over weekends, and she valued her personal time with her children too much to leave them to gaming on their own, and her boys were very busy children needing their exercise – a lot of what other professionals in the know (against gaming) are also saying.

So who to believe? What does it say when professional people developing and promoting games for your children, and grandchildren, will not allow them, or at least grossly restrict them, for their own children?

Back to gaming at large, we know that as part of their structure i-games are inherently entertaining, engaging, and emotionally rewarding: the most personalized form of entertainment and learning. However, in disagreement with Gee and others of his perspective, I believe there is no way that education can, or for that matter should, compete with this format. From my perspective the error here is that we are presuming that viewing and gaming formats are superior education modalities because of their ability to sustain or keep children's attention longer. Apart from studies that clearly challenge this position (e.g., Dr. Kuhl[116 117]), perhaps there are other errors in our thinking here? Perhaps our error is more basic, more fundamental, involving our increasing expectations of children to be able to sustain attention over longer and longer periods of time. Perhaps our error is in assuming that because a medium can extend an expectation, the original expectation should be surpassed.

> Our games, or screens, have to be a little bit boring; otherwise the brain does not learn to learn, it learns to be entertained.

I reference back to Chapter Three, when, in clinical practice, we too use games as therapeutic tools in neurotherapy to facilitate the learning of states of attention. Our games, or screens, have to be a little bit boring; otherwise the brain does not learn to learn, it learns to be entertained.

Seeking to continuously entertain children can backfire. When entertainment as opposed to learning becomes a primary or co-dependent goal of education, educators and parents will need to raise the bar over and over again as the novelty wears off. (Entertainment, in this scholastic context, is *not* to be confused with play). With this model children will need higher and higher levels of entertainment to keep them engaged in learning and play. Again full circle, inadvertently by permitting extensive viewing and gaming, we may be contributing to attention difficulties, behavioral regulation difficulties, and even depression. With all these childhood disorders on the rise, we may want to seriously consider the possible contribution of gaming and viewing to childhood pathology.

I am not arguing that we should not seek to interest children in or through novel and varied methods (as play itself involves), rather that we should be cautious regarding equating good teaching with entertaining teaching. Entertaining learning should be part of the learning diet, not the required staple. When equating good and bad teaching with entertaining and boring teaching, we risk not developing the skills necessary to sustain attention through the mundane aspects of life and learning alike. By entertaining constantly (in gaming, learning, and other activities) we may be creating a generation of bored thrill seekers who can no longer entertain themselves with self-initiated play and no longer learn under standard circumstances.

As will be discussed a little more in depth in the following chapter, to a certain extent this is already happening. Many educators I know have commented on the inability of the generation currently in the first and second year of university to sustain attention on longer segments of teaching: say, the three-hour lecture. Others have commented on the staccato of writing: how in essays paragraphs don't flow from one to another as if the young authors are incapable of sustaining a train of thought or concept past a certain figurative and literal space: what Prensky[118] spoke

By entertaining constantly (in gaming, learning, and other activities) we may be creating a generation of bored thrill seekers who can no longer entertain themselves with self-initiated play and no longer learn under standard circumstances.

of as preferred learning and writing style, and what I suspect is an adapted mind.

Many primary and high school children on the surface seem more intelligent; they know many snippets of science and historical trivia. Why do I call this trivia instead of knowledge? Apart from the scope itself being narrow, I am finding many children and young adults do not extend the knowledge. They do not integrate the information into broader concepts, theories, or philosophies. If individuals cannot do this, then indeed, trivia is all it remains: disconnected facts with no larger platform.

In sum, technologies, specifically i-tech modalities, are now dictating both conscious and unconscious changes in learning and now also memory. In my generation, I joke a little bit about how we all now carry a bit of our brains in our purses and pockets. Be it phone numbers, addresses, formulas, or facts, we memorize less and less. We don't have to: we open our phones and voilà!

The ability to see patterns and put pieces together is what larger or broader intelligence and later wisdom are based upon.

For the younger I am a little more concerned with the larger implications that instant access of information has on the broader scope of "non" learning: the potential marriage of "non" memorization to the "non" acquisition of knowledge. Fundamentally, we have to know something, and be able to reference it directly in our memory bank (in our brain, not our pocket) in order to integrate it or synthesize it with something else, with other knowledge. The ability to see patterns and put pieces together is what larger or broader intelligence and later wisdom are based upon. This is a little bit more than arguing the merits of entertaining versus non-entertaining learning platforms and related attention spans. It is also a primary underlying thesis of much of the work of Drs. Bauerlein and Carr amongst others. Would we realize how little we know if the Internet went down for a day?[119]

The larger question now is what are we learning and not learning? What are we truly facilitating with i-tech in the classroom?

Fabulous and Not So Fabulous Applications

One high school in my district has an extremely pro–i-tech stance. To this end they procured tablets for every one of their students, donated by a tech company. As part of the curriculum, every student was instructed to publish a daily blog. No insult to youth, but perhaps one percent of teenagers at this age have daily material worth publishing publicly to such a broad audience as their whole high school. Exploring this art is what a school newspaper (on- or offline) is for: semi-juried writings selected for their public interest.

For many the blogging exercise resembles more a public diary than any literary pondering: students telling of their days, and all the social-emotional consequences that come with them, including judgment of those who have interesting lives, flat lives, are more or less privileged based on what they do or don't do after school, or what they are or are not exposed to. In this public format, content can further, go offline, as well as to broader online networks such as Facebook.

With such an unstructured format, few adolescents become little philosophers. Few are reflecting on events or scenarios or integrating the learning from their daily lives. The format is also a little Orwellian, Big Brotherish: creepily voyeuristic and invasive. Adolescents, like all people, should be entitled to their privacy. Classmates, teachers, and principals should have no right to demand knowledge of, or be able to access many components of one's personal life (unless they feel a child is in emotional or physical peril). By definition personal life is personal! I haven't even approached the major pitfalls of uncensored or unstructured blogging such as the promotion of confabulating sensationalist writings or the spiral blog[120]: both rather bad news in adolescence.

Now It Is Not All Bad...

In contrast, there are magnificent applications: ones that use Gee's principles, such as a high school in the Boston region which organized a community project wherein i-tech was central to its success (Community PlanIt,[121] if anyone cares to look it up). This project involved true investigation, including the collection and consolidation of information, and dissemination of information thereafter. It involved the students planning and strategizing, reflecting and integrating information as well as the learning of true teamwork, personal responsibility, and the acquisition of technical computer skills. The list goes on.

So as I repeat, it ain't all bad, not at all. But we cannot blindly accept or blindly apply the technologies without looking at the larger picture. We need to know specifically what we want to accomplish with i-media and i-tech applications and thereafter construct the relevant structure to facilitate the educational or scholastic objectives. No delusions here either: to do it right, a lot of deliberation and thought has to go into project development long before the children or students are involved. Arguably, when done right, i-tech is not faster or easier at all. And, as with all curriculum, with i-curriculum one needs to know what one wishes to accomplish with the tool. Equally one needs to know, or foresee, the potential pitfalls.

> We need to know specifically what we want to accomplish with i-media and i-tech applications and thereafter construct the relevant structure to facilitate the educational or scholastic objectives.

The lessons all seem to point in one direction: when i-tech replaces human interaction, whether instruction from a teacher or parent, play or interaction with a friend, it not only loses its advantage, it turns bad. i-tech should be an addition, an augment, a facilitator not a replacement for what we can deliver each other.

Delivery and Recording Systems: The Pen and the Keyboard.

Now that I have discussed the educational delivery system and placed it under some relative scrutiny, what of the recording system?

Keyboarding is fast replacing traditional longhand writing or scribing. Some argue it is vastly more efficient. In many regards it is. Indeed all i-tech platforms that support keyboarding are largely responsible for the great and entirely positive dissemination and sharing of information: social, political, educational, and otherwise. Documents are now completely transportable by all mediums to all places at all times. In the positive, digital natives are as a result arguably most politically and socially aware, and act accordingly. But keyboarding and the associated delivery format are changing a little more than accessibility: they are arguably changing the way we think, or should I say, the way we process our thoughts.

We are now processing differently based on the tools we use. I don't think there is necessarily any right or wrong here; it's just different, and I merely ask that we note such difference. We should also note that we are still in transition.

Keyboarding Versus Scribing – What Our Tools Do to Thinking

Scribing (printing or cursive longhand) requires synthesis in the mind; we pause before we write. As children we physically have to learn how to slow down our brains to get ideas to paper. Learning to scribe is an exercise in learning how to simultaneously pace the speed of thought with the speed, or learning of, functional motor skills.

When we write, a thought must be finished, actually thought out, before we set pen to paper to record it. Yes, we may edit in first, second, and even third drafts before we get to final copy, but with the pen, this stage is more a polishing of ideas than a formation or a processing of them. When we keyboard, in contrast, we purge, we just get the idea(s) out. We then return. We return to not only spell-check, correct typos, structure, and grammar; we return to actually (re)formulate, to sculpt the ideas themselves on the screen. Again, nothing wrong with this: it's just significantly different from scribing as a creative as well as a mental process.

That said, we may not want to abandon scribing entirely. As I say to many parents, do have your child keyboard in school and elsewhere, but make sure that one recording format, or rather processing format, does not completely supersede the other. Not yet. Indeed the world is changing, but just like language in bicultural regions, functioning with one fewer language can put a person at a severe cultural, social, scholastic, and yes, intellectual disadvantage.

Educational Oversights

Today, many children who keyboard early and do not learn writing, or rather thinking or processing structure by pen, suddenly find they are completely derailed by pen and paper exams or tests that require sentences or paragraphs (or God-forbid essays) as responses. These children and young adults then get special learning disability designations, permission to have scribes, or the privilege of oral examinations as opposed to written ones. Yet another learning disability is emerging, Written Output Disorder, and/or various processing disorders. From my clinical perspective, for the vast majority of children, these disorders are not learning disabilities at all. They are due to a critical educational oversight. In our eagerness to advance, we are not adequately preparing students for the multiple modalities they still require to function in our current school culture. We have failed these children in our expectations. Today's students still need to learn how to function in two modalities, two currencies or languages. Continuing with the language analogy: we are telling, or teaching, children it is just fine to learn only how to write in English, and then we turn around and give them a test in Greek.

Again, such shifts are not new, nor are they negative. Not so very long ago, arguably, we were not even a literate species. We became progressively literate with the invention of the printing press and the resulting dissemination of writings to the masses as opposed to the educated elite. Thereafter, with education policies, we gradually shifted from an oral culture to a written culture. In the majority of Western societies, stories, maps, and lessons are now delivered by print rather than song or oral story. That said, because we learned how to read and write, acquired books, newspapers, and song sheets, we did not forget how to sing, or preach, listen or tell stories by the campfire.

To Process or Not to Process

In our zeal to accept the new recording system we must not forget the processing system, meaning we still need to process and format our thoughts somewhere: if not in our heads, then on our screens. It is simply a matter of where and how, not if or if not, we should do it. This, I believe, is a primary complaint of educators that unfortunately gets trapped in the anti-digital argument. I do not believe these educators have any issue whatsoever with the digital mode itself; they have issue with its caveat: the incomplete method.

In the digital age, we must be careful not to succumb to the "instantness," what I referred to as the "purge" or stage one. We must ensure we teach the young to progress to stage two. They too must be taught to regulate themselves to not be satisfied with first thought. In the end it is not so different. There is an educational process to learning how to keyboard as there is to learning how to scribe. Somewhere we, the educators, forgot this; perhaps we too were mesmerized by the method, and forgot that the purpose of all writing regardless of method is communication, and, when learned well, artistry.

We should also recall that some old ways remain good ways, and should not be completely forsaken for the new. Case in point, many of us, although quite literate, succeed best in remembering things if we put them into ditties or to song. This is now being (re) introduced as a "new" learning method. Not new at all (pre-literacy), it was the primary method for centuries.

Confounding Principles

Another thing to keep in mind is the ease with which we can confuse method and context. There are definitively different contexts or voices to keyboarding, or should I say key tapping. Texting is rather like talking (except it leaves a record). Indeed we do just purge and send, and here appropriately so, due to context. Have you ever read transcribed speech? It is eye-opening how many "errors" we make when speaking. So why do we, the older, expect refining from the new "speech" modality? (This indeed is a hang-up of many of my digital immigrant generation.) In texting, we also use the new contractions or txt talk, arguably a new language itself. This indeed is a generational divide, one wherein one generation will dictate to another what is proper or not (e.g., "u r" is not acceptable in a university essay, but write however you wish socially, e.g., on Facebook). Until that generation is old enough to rewrite the rules, that is (pun intended ☺) In the meantime, we follow established practice and keep the debate going (e.g., is text talk acceptable in business email or just social email, what about in a quick memo?). Here too we owe it to the young to remain conscious of potential educational oversights. If they are not explicitly taught context, we cannot accuse children and youth of ignorance.

> ...it is all about the processing. When we take notes by keyboard apparently we process at a much shallower level. Many of us don't even process at all.

Now all that said, in the keyboarding versus scribing debate, a few studies clearly indicate that we (all of us young and old) remember more, and significantly more, by writing than by keyboarding. Again it is all about the processing. When we take notes by keyboard apparently we process at a much shallower level. Many of us don't even process at all. We type verbatim as opposed to selecting key concepts or words for later recall. We record as opposed to learn.[122] For students, or those who need to memorize or otherwise shelve information in brain memory, as opposed to digital banks, the implication is, we must go over our typed notes as if new. When we scribe, it appears we have already retained something in the process.

We also must be careful to not get ahead of our brain wiring. In the keyboarding versus scribing debate, the jury is still out, but currently weighing in toward the need for some continued kinetic involvement in learning. The scribing of letters (both cursive and printing) has been directly associated with later success at learning how to read. It appears that children who learn keyboarding exclusively are later significantly compromised at letter recognition, and hence reading.[123] This may be as simple as pattern recognition; "making it" equals learning it (a fundamental component of experiential learning theory). It also ties in a lot with my clinical work involving EEG brainwaves and learning disabilities. Compromised Sensory Motor Rhythm (SMR, a 13 to 15Hz brainwave) is associated with learning disorders. We often train Sensory Motor Rhythm for written output disorders as well as compromised reading abilities. In fact, a lot of the early work on ADHD involved sensorimotor brainwaves, not just inattentive (Theta) brainwaves. SMR was a primary focus of ADD and ADHD research as far back as the late 1970s.[124] [125] In sum, engaging motor skills appears to be married to pattern recognition and thereafter functional meaning and larger learning (including maintaining focus as well as specific skills such as reading and writing).

The larger implication is in our eagerness to accept the new, we risk not seeing the larger picture: how the neural networks (or the dots of our brains) connect for learning. The very young, as well as those in very active learning phases, such as students, can be grossly affected by our oversights.

Elders, educators, researchers, policy makers, professionals, and yes, parents too, have a social responsibility to not forget to look at methods or processes of absorption as dictated by methods of delivery before we teach them, give them, or sell them, to those who are naive.

Going back to studies alluded to earlier, it seems we also remember more, learn more, and tremendously more from human delivery than from i-tech or screen delivery. This is explicitly due to variation in human interactive process as well as broader environmental attention. The effects are black and white in the very young. Babies, although attentively watching screens, learn absolutely nothing from programs.[126] Many even learn less[127] than those perceived as doing nothing at all (e.g., sitting gazing out of their cradles or highchairs). With babies in particular, there is no such thing as doing nothing. They are learning incredible amounts from observation: seeing, hearing, touching, feeling, mimicking, and playing.[128]

I have been speaking a lot about children, students, and the very young. It appears these effects are not exclusive to young minds at all. A growing market for educational or cognitive i-tech games is the older, even the elder. Many gaming products are now exclusively marketed to adults. Promoting brain exercises based in principles of neuroplasticity, they proclaim gains in cognitive flexibility, superior intelligence, and a defense against cognitive decline. I first was rather supportive. In contrast to children, it appeared cognitive games for individuals over forty much like Sudoku and crossword puzzles helped keep the brain active and were therefore beneficial, or at least not harmful.

Similar to gaming for children and the Baby Einstein craze, however, there appears to be a lot of smoke and shadows behind the claims. A meta-analysis of studies[129] found slight improvements in the ability to remember visual images and the ability to remember recent events but no changes in planning or judgment abilities nor attention or selective concentration abilities (otherwise known as executive function, or the brain function that regulates larger cognitive function). Also rather ironic, the more you use the games, the less they work; more than three sessions a week was associated with decline, not improvement. Again, this may not be a function of what the games are or are not doing, but what people are not doing when choosing to game (e.g., they are not socializing, exercising, or partaking in other healthy activities but rather staying in isolation training with i-devices). Further, less than thirty minutes proved ineffective, and home sessions as opposed to, you got it, supervised or class sessions were ineffective. So is it again the personal or social element, the community element, that is the key variable to success?

For adults, I, for one, am going to recommend we honor the Boot, Blakely and Simons thesis.[130] Until further research shows otherwise, don't buy into the educational hype and play i-games to improve cognitive function; play them if you enjoy them, play them if you think they are fun. But not too much...

CHAPTER EIGHT

From i-Kids to i-Brains

In this chapter I would like to speak to my greater concern. Not changes in temporary brain state(s), or vulnerabilities that leave us all somewhat liable, not even the differences in integration of the different i-generations, or the strengths and weaknesses of delivery and processing methods, but rather the risk of irreversible changes in brain function that we now suspect may be interfering with the brain development of the very young.

The younger are now experiencing particular risks and effects that the older are not. In this chapter I am going to explore what I refer to as full assimilation of digital media: not in the positive form of integration, or even negative interference, but rather a brain rewiring. Think The Borg.

Now that you have that creepy *Star Trek* image in your head, it is not far off. In its extreme, there is mounting evidence that the early introduction of digital media is irreversibly changing the brains of infants in most critical phases of development, making them orient more toward objects than people.

On a lighter note it is making them a little more stupid; more politely put, it is thwarting learning. Back to the heavier note, it is affecting social development at its core; it is affecting attachment. Very young children are starting to relate to technologies and objects more than with parents and caregivers, and this can have irreversible affects in both socialization and emotional deregulation. It is also a key symptom of Autism.

i-Pad in the Cradle

I was recently out for dinner at a lovely French bistro when a group of diners caught my attention. The group consisted of three young couples and a child I would guess was somewhere between the age of eighteen months and two years. As they settled in, it was evident that this child was extremely well behaved, happy in his highchair at the end of the table. My first thoughts were "how lovely" that these young parents were including their child in their adult outing as opposed to leaving him home with a babysitter or going to a child-centered restaurant earlier in the day. The true notion of inclusion: somewhat lost in today's increasingly polarized child-centered versus child-exclusive culture. And then they pulled out a tablet.

For one in my profession what came next was very sad to watch. As the mother set up the tablet for the child, he was watching her. He was not at all interested in the tablet. Five minutes later he still was not interested. He was looking around the restaurant and then to his mother. He looked at the objects on the table and at the faces around the table. After each scanning, he would try to make contact with one or both of his parents; he would reach up toward them a bit, focus on them a while. He was seeking the attention, and social reinforcement, of his parents. The saddest thing was that his parents never looked back. They were engaged with their friends, and only their friends. The inevitable happened: the child then engaged with the tablet, exactly as intended.

What concerns me most here is this child was not at all "disturbing." It was evident that the occasional glance, smile, or touch of a parent would have sufficed: this child was completely capable of self-entertaining with the occasional parental reinforcement. In my professional terminology, he was completely regulated.

So why was I so disturbed?

Because everything *was* perfect...prior to the tablet, and prior to his parents disengaging from him, that is. Everything I saw in this child himself pointed to healthy development including healthy attachment. He was curious about his environment and connected to his parents. He was attached, engaged, emotionally regulated, and very well behaved.

Redirecting Development

What we are learning is when parents substitute their attention with digital media under these "perfect" circumstances, they essentially risk triggering a process of brain rewiring: a process that has great potential to thwart critical phases of development.

By directing the child to a tablet, parents change the child's orientation from observation of people and the larger environment, and seeking their approval, to the extremely narrow focus on an object and its content. If this is the way this young couple intends to continue to parent, this is the way the brain will start to rewire. This is the making of an i-brain.

Substituting Ourselves – Reconditioning Children Toward Objects and Peers

When parents substitute i-tech for themselves when a very young child is seeking their engagement, they will begin to recondition the child's social, emotional, and later cognitive development. The child will start to be conditioned toward the tablet (and other digital media) as opposed to people. When we change orientation and ignore a child in social environments, the child will quickly adapt, learning to orient toward what we give him.

First learning, then knowing that he is not included, the child from the restaurant will soon be asking for the tablet in social environments either verbally, or by acting out. In little time this will develop into his preference. By choice, he will not want so much to engage with adults anymore (and perhaps not even other children) but rather with the tablet. When a little older, and not directly entertained, he will most likely even start consistently pestering for an i-tech device to entertain him. The long-term effect is it will thwart his social learning and his social interaction.

This conditioning will also likely affect emotional regulation. Directing such a well-regulated child to i-tech and then ignoring him risks destabilization. The child will note the systematic rejection by his primary caretaker(s) and soon learn to auto-regulate (feel better) with technology, not people.

The child will note the systematic rejection by his primary caretaker(s) and soon learn to auto-regulate (feel better) with technology, not people.

People, his people, are not paying attention to him anyway. Note this child originally did not want the tablet; he wanted to "be there." He will learn to want the tablet through the primary emotion of rejection, not of interest or of intrigue.

Healthy Patterns

The usual natural and healthy pattern of children is to explore and check in, explore and check in: exactly what this little fellow was instinctually doing. Infants and later children do this check-in for approval (including the learning of physical and emotional safety), as well as for inclusion. This starts very early. Little babies grab something and look up; little children run to the edge of the pool and yell "look at me" before jumping. As children get older, the circle of exploration widens. They either physically go further away, or deeper into an activity, and will check in once in an afternoon for said approval as opposed to once every fifteen seconds or fifteen minutes. Sometime in their teens, most start experimenting with not checking in: no longer wanting or seeking parental approval. The cycle is complete.

Developmental Intention: Imprinting and Attachment

There is a natural developmental purpose to all this: the baby looking up after grabbing something will get a nod of approval or a frown stating this does not make the parent happy. The little one yelling at the edge of the pool will get smiling eyes, a thumbs-up, or a call of "careful, the water is shallow" and reorient their action accordingly. This holds for learning state regulation as well. A child that falls will start to cry, and often continue or stop based not on the level of pain or hurt they feel but rather on parental reaction. There is an incredible amount of environmental, emotional, and social learning going on in this pattern of parent-child engagement. And the child wants it, is seeking it! Note it is not full-on play, not full-on attention, but rather just being there, being aware.

I know a lot more about people than animals. That said, much like animals imprint, humans attach, and human attachment is very fragile in human psychosocial development.

Being "Not There"

Maté and Neufeld[131] wrote a wonderful book wherein they referred to the eroding of generational hierarchy: how parenting was becoming increasingly difficult as children were orienting to peers as opposed to parents and elders. This is in part why. We are partially at fault: by providing i-media to distract them to free ourselves, we are also orienting away from them. We are substituting i-media for ourselves. The outcome we are now experiencing is that children first orient toward media and objects, then to peers, and lastly to parents.

Why Is Parental Orientation So Important?

When parental presence is less readily available and appears less important, children will turn elsewhere for what they need. This means they will get both their approval and their lessons elsewhere, including behavioral influence. And when children no longer look to parents to orient their behavior and emotions, they are reduced to instinct and impulse.[132] In this state, they make decisions to jump or not jump without any prior "learned" knowledge transferred from their parents and caregivers. *See the true and now negative ADHD connection?*

In the case of the five-second verbal exchange above regarding jumping by the pool, the message from the parent could transfer caution, confidence, or both – all presumably absorbed, acted on, and banked for future reference when a parent is no longer in visual range or earshot.

Children need to turn somewhere and without this initial guardian set-up, they will increasingly look to messages from media and peers. They are turning to equally socially and developmentally immature and emotionally irresponsible peers as opposed to responsible mature adults for models of how to behave.[133] They are also turning to messages received from media: screenwriters, gaming programmers, and marketers with a vested interest in manipulating children's behavior, desires, and guiding their (your) purchases.[134] [135] [136]

With perceived parental unavailability, children also become emotionally deregulated: they become stoic or emotionally unavailable, or contrarily, very needy. They cry with a fall not because the fall itself hurts, but because there was no one to soothe, protect, or even acknowledge them when it happened. Perceived absence is where the pain comes from, where anxiety comes from. It is the foundation of the notion of absence of social support.

And now, the science behind this.

Attachment Theory 101

Parent-baby face-to-face or heart-to-heart engagement forms the core of the social engagement system from which the child and later adult will function in all subsequent relationships. It is physically setting up bidirectional neuronal communication, otherwise referred to as brain wiring. Face-to-face interaction (as well as touch) is the portal by which brain systems learn the regulation of psychological state including safety, happiness, fear, and anxiety.[137]

As humans we are wired to learn this way. Infants are genetically programmed to connect with caregivers. This connection, referred to as attachment, is a biologically programmed adaptive system that drives development itself. When the attachment system fails, through failed interaction (lack of touch or focus through vocal or facial expression), the child's development is affected. Minor variations result in variation in attachment style (e.g., minor anxious attachment, such as clingy people, or minor disorganized attachment, such as slightly socially awkward people). Major variations, resulting in faulty or insecure attachment, result in halted or alternate development and pathology (AKA true blue mental illness). In the extreme, an alternate process coined "neuronal Darwinism" development halts as neuronal pathways that would normally be activated via caregiver interaction do not form. In the nature-nurture dynamic, nature will not develop if not nurtured. At this very tender young age, brain wiring or brain development will alter.[138] [139] [140] [141] [142]

What Happens When We Are "Not" There

Violations of the expected attention of a caretaker shift body physiology, which means when we don't follow the expected rules of care, the child will not follow the expected rules of stability. A little being's developing nervous system will change from a state of calm to a state of defense such as fear and anxiety (e.g., the little fellow who falls will feel anxious not because he is actually hurt but because he feels there is no one to protect him if he were truly hurt). Conversely little children will stop crying when we tell them or otherwise show them they are okay; equally, if we express over-concern, so will they.

Difficulties regulating state (controlled by our nervous system) are the core to the later development of behavioral problems in children and later psychiatric disorders in adolescence and adulthood.[143] In infancy, the physiological system is confirming wiring paths or neuronal connections associated with environments, emotions, and people/relationships.

Back to my little story in the restaurant, in the absence of the tablet, if the parents just ignored the child long enough he would eventually cry or tantrum; a little being becomes completely destabilized when ignored so in a new environment. He would gradually become terrified (requiring much settling and soothing thereafter). This need not mean a parent's attention must always be on the child; indeed this is not recommended either (as we see in the helicopter parenting phenomenon, such a child will deregulate for other reasons). What is important is that parents "repair" their absence (when paying attention to others or something else for any extended amount of time). That they physically check in once in a while with positive eye contact, a smile, vocalization, or a touch, letting the child in turn know he or she is safe. If the parent has not been "gone" too long, many adjusted children will settle and be happy to go back to observation or play post said check-in; they will learn to self-entertain and explore their little world in these feelings of safety. They will also need progressively less and less attention because of the solid development of this concept of safety. Attachment is a two-way street, with both the child and the parent occasionally, yet consistently, checking in.(Note: Checking in should not be confused with helicopter parenting or the tiger/ dragon mom phenomenon; these parenting styles are grounded in over-observance and over-control. Again the check-in involves being available rather than truly present or occupied with the child. The developmental purpose of the check-in is the development of autonomy in secure attachment.)

Cancelling Information

The issue with i-media is the magic combination of absence of parent (figurative or literal) and substitution with media. The giving of an iPod, phone, or a tablet is very different than the giving of jingling keys, a soother, or a stuffy. Why? Simply put, none of the other toys or objects cancels out the larger environment.

The majority of learning at this age comes from observation (followed later by physical exploration); infants and toddlers look both proximally and later distally at the faces and expressions around them, at the objects near them, and listen to sounds before they become words. They listen to the sing-song of happiness versus the staccato of anger, otherwise known as voice prosody. In this interaction, children learn notions of safety and security, as well as danger, from parents and caregivers. For example, if the child in the restaurant observed an angry man at the next table, the smiling face of his mother would still make him feel safe. If the man started to raise his voice and his mother tensed in response, the child would learn danger associated with a stranger yelling, not necessarily from the voice tone of the man himself, but rather from the tensing of his mother. The same might occur if the little fellow reached for his father's steak knife and started to pull it to his mouth and his mother took it away and replaced it with a spoon. Her facial expression or voice prosody would have denoted danger or fear while noticing the knife, followed by some positive expression or tone when removing it and/or replacing it with the spoon. With i-media the child is learning none of this, not safety, not security, not danger, nor threat, nor exploration of all of the aforementioned. And definitely not the delicate balance one's "people," and later community (first parents, then friends, and later partners), provide in the delicate protective dynamic in all of the above.

The primary concern with the early introduction of i-tech is that it directly thwarts interactive developmental process between parent and child. When i-tech is in use, parents and children dramatically reduce, if not stop, the interactive process responsible for triggering the development of neuronal connections (or brain wiring) necessary for attachment, which in turn lays the foundation for all subsequent socio-emotional development. Point blank, both parent and child stop checking in. The child becomes mesmerized and rarely looks up. The parent, knowing this, thereafter rarely looks down.

The primary concern with the early introduction of i-tech is that it directly thwarts interactive developmental process between parent and child.

Changing Our Perception and Our Learning

Some interesting earlier studies explore the effect of media in what I refer to as the cancelling of social-emotional information as well as non-specific or environmental learning. The first comes from a study on inoculations. It appears that the viewing of media not only completely enthralls us, as outlined in previous chapters, it does so to such a degree that it acts as an analgesic (a pain killer or sedative). i-tech is strong stuff!

Not Learning Emotion

In a study on pain perception, children who were distracted by watching a screen as opposed to being distracted by or engaging with their mothers during vaccination, reported significant reduction in the perception of pain.[144] The head author of this study speculated that viewing may be functioning as an analgesic or pacifier by obscuring the intake of other information, in this case the transfer of emotion. He speculated that as the children's attention was on the screen, they were not paying attention to or even aware of the emotions around them. Specifically, when viewing, children cannot or do not perceive their mother's underlying empathy for pain or fear regarding the vaccination. The children are not picking up on their mother's subtle or unintentional transfer of affect (emotion) underlying her attempts at entertainment and distraction from the vaccination (from the pain of the needle). Essentially, the viewing of a screen overrides the ability to read subtle emotional cues in a child's immediate environment. This too may have implications in the development of autistic characteristics.

Reducing Learning Efficiency

Screen viewing at a very young age also affects larger learning. Studies on preschoolers have found a connection between early television viewing and the development of attention disorders. Television viewing at age one and age three have both been associated with a marked increased risk of developing ADHD at age seven.[145] Television is also associated with problems in behavioral and affective regulation[146] [147]and sleep disturbance.[148] Earlier, I also spoke of second language acquisition studies wherein babies paying full attention to a person via a screen, as compared to by a person next to them, learned absolutely nothing.[149] Of note, other studies have found lesser relationships between viewing and attention difficulties or learning. In my view such studies tend to speak to the compounding effect rather than the null effect of the viewing process. The number of hours one watches in childhood tends to be directly related to attention difficulties in adolescence completely independent of budding attention difficulties evident in early childhood.[150] Translation: nothing wrong with a little TV or i-media, a lot wrong with a lot.

> Translation: nothing wrong with a little TV or i-media, a lot wrong with a lot.

Dual Delusions

This leads to the second dual delusion touched on in previous chapters: that not only is viewing not harmful (developmentally and otherwise), but that it is educational. Contrary, my friends: for infants, programs marketed for their educational value, such as (of all names) the Baby Einstein series, have been found to have the exact opposite effect. Zimmerman, Christakis, and Meltzoff[151] found that in infants eight to sixteen months of age, the hours spent watching "educational" videos and television intended to expand infants' vocabularies did quite the opposite. For every hour spent viewing, infants understood between six and eight fewer words than infants with lesser exposure. What's happening?

Back to the baby in the restaurant: engaging with a tablet may not be explicitly making him or other infants not learn; rather, as the researchers above suspected, watching a screen, regardless of content, eclipses other opportunities to learn. When infants are watching a screen they are not actively interacting with a caregiver. They are not being played with, read to, sung to, or even looked at. Nor are they looking around, observing, listening, and being curious. Essentially their cognitive and emotional learning is limited to the specific content explicitly "being taught" by the program or screen. Educational videos and programming either restrict or reduce learning as they substitute for interactive environments that are conducive to broader integrative or full learning as well as development.[152] In sum, they narrow us.

It is not what the viewing itself is doing, but rather what is *not* happening in the developmental cycle, while the infant, preschooler, and later young child is engaged with the medium.

Many studies finding that viewing is associated with cognitive and affective disorders (learning and emotional problems) are completely in keeping with developmental theory. It is not what the viewing itself is doing, but rather what is *not* happening in the developmental cycle, while the infant, preschooler, and later young child is engaged with the medium. The hours spent in front of viewing devices, as opposed to contact with caregivers and the global environment, may have a compounding effect on development by interrupting the progression of developmental systems that are activated by caregiver interaction: full circle back to attachment theory.

Scientific Corner: Developmental Theory: The way infants are supported in the initial months of life is key to how they will develop and interact with others later in life (Rayner, Joyce, Rose, Twyman, and Clulow, 2005).[153] When children are viewing, as opposed to interacting with caregivers (parents or otherwise), for large portions of their infancy and early childhood, it may alter the way development is programmed. This is consistent with the writings of the heavy hitters in developmental and attachment theory, namely Learner, Schore, and Bowlby. In sum, viewing will affect all subsequent relationships.

Bowlby (1969/1982),[154] in his seminal work on attachment theory, established the critical role of parental interaction and subsequent development of effective regulation. Neurobiologically, brain structures responsible for the mediation of emotional (including social) functioning are rapidly developing in early infancy and appear to be directly related to the quality of caregiver interaction. When specific events, experiences, and interactions with caregivers do not occur (or do not occur with sufficient frequency), they directly affect development on a neuronal level leading to variance in in brain development and hence behavior (Shore, 2001).[155] Behavior, and cognitive and social development, are all based on dynamic interaction with initial attachment (Lerner, 1985).[156] In sum, initial attachment and interaction with caregivers is the foundation for healthy development, period. Consistent consumption of i-media distorts and rewires this.

Bottom line, you don't want your infants to not learn or reduce their learning due to i-media. You also do not want your children to attach to an object other than a blanket in bed, a teddy bear, or a doll (which serve temporary roles in positive socio-emotional substitution and the learning of self-soothing). You will also note that healthy children grow out of attachment with dolls and stuffy objects, and non-cuddly toys have natural interest cycles. Pardon the constant sub-referencing to Autism, but again hyper-focus on a specific toy or subject that a child does not mature out of (or for that matter *into*, e.g., an obsession with dinosaurs leading to a career in paleontology) is again a classic symptom of the disorder. Back to i-tech, most non-tech games and toys tend to be noncompetitive with caregiver attachment, serving their own role in mimicking, creative play, and even strategy development.

CHAPTER NINE

Learning, Play, and Parenting: Conflicting Needs in a Busy, Busy World

Why Is This Happening?

Now that I have explored what is happening vis-à-vis young children's socio-emotional development, early parenting, and i-tech, I will explore some of the reasons why: why we are embracing mass consumption and early introduction of i-media for children. With a little walk through history, and a little more developmental theory, I will explore larger cultural shifts in parenting and family systems, expand on the blurred lines of learning and play, and look at the not-so-clear differences between what I believe are healthy versus unhealthy applications of i-tech in play and education.

Let's Talk Truth

Apart from consumer naiveté, misinformation, and conflicting information from industry and services, there is a buy-in factor. Why are we – parents, teachers, and educators at large – buying in?

Most parents are not bad parents, and most teachers are not lazy. Most elders really want the best for youth, so why are we embracing the components of i-media that are evidently harmful?

Why are we literally buying and otherwise facilitating excessive access to i-tech to children?

Family Systems and Cultural Change

The Big Shift

Over the past fifty years, the family has undergone considerable changes. Parenting is changing, and dramatically so. For starters, parental work duties and financial and material expectations for "providing" are increasing at the same time support systems for young families are diminishing. There is significantly more running around, less parent-child interaction, and higher stress and fatigue of parent(s) when one-on-one time does occur.[157] [158] So who, or should I say "what," has filled the gap? You got it: i-media.

The simple answer is i-media is acting as a stress and fatigue mediator for parents. We embrace it because is it filling a need, and now a void. Engagement with digital media requires little to no pre-planning, is instantly available, and provides parents, caretakers, and even educators with much needed moments of respite and solace.

It is more than likely that the parents in my little restaurant story were trying to preempt a tantrum or other by setting up the tablet. Perhaps they had not been out with these friends since the birth of the child and were desperate for some adult interaction. The tablet was their way of ensuring all went well so they could have some non–baby time themselves. In sum, the tablet would ensure the baby and his needs would not be in conflict with parental needs by his needs taking over the dinner and the otherwise adult interaction.

How Did This Happen?

As the family and its needs shifted, multimedia was popularly perceived as a tool facilitating parenting. The otherwise inquisitive, noisy, or fighting children in the back seat of the car were quiet, first with a DVD and now with an iPad or iPhone.

A single working mother can take a shower, dress herself, and prepare for work by placing her infant child in front of cartoons or any digital screen. A parent can engage with a service person, make an appointment at the doctors', or chat with a neighbor by handing a pestering child her iPhone. A couple can debrief, do the laundry uninterrupted, and perhaps, if lucky, have a few moments to themselves as their children engross themselves in gaming. Such are the realities of modern parenting. In our frantic pace of life, digital media is perceived as the most efficient and perhaps most cost-effective babysitter since grandma. Why? Because parents are too darned busy and no longer have social or functional support.

> ...parents are too darned busy and no longer have social or functional support.

Traditional nuclear families with localized extended family units are less and less common. We moved away from our own towns and parents, many of us are single parents, few of us know our neighbors well enough to request assistance never mind entrust our children to them, and the remaining aunties, uncles, and grandmas and grandpas got dethroned, went on strike, moved away themselves, or are equally busy. Someone, or "something," had to fill the parenting gap.

The Electronic Babysitter

To this end, the medium can completely capture a child or children's attention for much-needed moments of parental reprieve. Parents use the medium as an electronic babysitter, believing that it is both educational and entertaining for their children. The catch however is that while i-tech may be providing temporary reprieve, it simultaneously and cumulatively is rendering other aspects of parenting and family life more difficult.

As mentioned in previous chapters, excessive and early application of i-tech in childhood misaligns attachment (including

Over time, the medium does exactly the opposite of what we wish: it actually revs children up and emotionally deregulates them, leaving them more likely to tantrum and less capable of self-entertaining, self-occupying.

emotional regulation) and affects development. Over time, the medium does exactly the opposite of what we wish: it actually revs children up and emotionally deregulates them, leaving them more likely to tantrum and less capable of self-entertaining, self-occupying. It also affects their ability to sustain focus in school and on homework, self-care, parental direction, or chores. In sum, it affects their efficiency at both their "jobs" (schooling and chores) as well as their "off time" AKA, play, as well as their emotional stability. The medium so very, very ironically renders children more demanding of time in a world where parents are increasingly pressed for time, resulting in reducing the pleasures and amplifying the notion of burden in parenthood.

Knowing this, and seeing this as a practicing therapist, I am terrified by the current marketing practice of explicitly pandering i-tech products to fatigued, stressed-out, or otherwise occupied and unavailable parents: products such as the Nova-Pad that literally promote the ability of a product "to occupy any child throughout the day." Now that bulletins are out on the potentially devastating effects of i-tech before the age of two,[159] business is marketing to the next catchment group (three- to six-year-olds), precisely the children in the next critical phases of development post attachment – the phases wherein cognitive-behavioral learning is set up and socio-emotional foundations are solidified – developmental phases wherein, once again, the presence of parents, vested caretakers, and/or others of one's people is needed "throughout the day"!

Two pro-tech for toddlers arguments I often hear, and wish to address directly, are: one, active therapists, such as myself, only see deregulated children and it distorts our perspective; and two, digital immigrants are holding to the realities of their generation(s) and are subsequently blind to change they do not understand or partake in, and are thus biased against progress and said change.

When hearing these counter-arguments, I appeal to all parents, professionals, educators, and policy makers to not dismiss decades of research on attachment, developmental and learning theory, neurology, and brain wiring already presented for the flash and apparent ease of i-tech. Human interaction in the early phases of human development remains critical. Indeed, the weaker (or neurologically liable) fall sooner, and problems are always first evidenced in clinical populations. Parallel issues, however, are also now being noted in the non-clinical population (those not in active treatment). We are truly in a live experiment, and, until we definitely know the outcome, we owe it to ourselves and to the generations that follow to keep our eyes open and be cautious with young little brains and lives. Second, to hear the battle hymn and not to fall for the red herring: what most of us are saying is a) nothing wrong with a little, a lot wrong with a lot (e.g., "occupying a child throughout the day") and b) nothing wrong with assimilation, a lot wrong with an override. Meaning, use i-tech, all i-tech freely and wisely as a tool to accompany human purpose and human pleasure but not as a total replacement for human interaction (in education, play, sexuality, communication, caregiving, etc.).

External Extra-Attitudinal Burdens

Unfortunately it does not end here, and we can't blame all the difficulties of modern parenting on i-tech. Many cultural factors and, I must also say, capitalistic interests currently intensify the perceived duties of parenting and by proxy the burden of parenting. Three prime contributors are media, law, and business venture.

Danger, Danger Everywhere

The first major negative influence I believe is tightly linked with the fear-mongering practice of news media and, by proxy, community.

Media blasts all and everything negative, making us focus on these negatives, magnifying natural and healthy parental fears regarding the safety and security of their children to unnatural and unhealthy dimensions.

What we are being shown and told by media is now making us feel irresponsible and afraid to send our children alone or in the company of siblings or other kids to the woods behind our homes, the city park down the street, or to the free swim at the lifeguarded swimming pool by bus. So instead we drive them and wait, increasing our own parental burden, or we settle them with i-tech. Of note, check your local statistics on accidents and crimes against children. In most communities, you will probably find the world is actually safer now for children than it was in the 1950s. It is just when something goes terribly wrong, and don't get me wrong, it occasionally does, it is blasted everywhere, making us equally believe that the perils themselves are everywhere.

Broken Bones Versus Broken Minds

Along with deafening cries of parental irresponsibility, if you are not monitoring your child at every moment when they wish to climb out of the nest and start exploring, there is also a rather new and equally frightening fact called legal liability. Children's environments including playgrounds and parks are getting significantly more "safe" and, I might add, less interesting. This is our fault, as we are increasingly placing responsibility on others – suing people, organizations, community centers, and the city – rather than looking at ourselves and how we educate our children vis-à-vis safety and play. In reaction, community is increasingly protecting itself.

The park across the street from my old home recently removed the zip line on which there were hours and hours of fun to be had. Why? Because children could hurt themselves. Of course they can; they can also hurt themselves by climbing trees, riding bikes, jumping on trampolines, swinging on swings, pogo sticks, skateboards, and all the wonderful games and adventures of childhood.

As outlined in previous chapters, this is part of it all, the learning of actual boundaries: the dangers and risks of our physical limitations, and of adventure itself.

Adventure and the Learning of Boundaries

Ironically by playing more and more exclusively on i-devices and in virtual as opposed to actual realities, children are no longer learning physical or for that matter emotional boundaries. They are simultaneously over-fearful and under-fearful (far too anxious and reactive as well as far too impulsive). We have fewer and fewer children who are calculated as opposed to avoidant or impulsive risk takers. Calculated as opposed to impulsive risk taking, by the way, is a clear boundary between extraordinary success and failure in much of personal and professional life thereafter.

A very interesting study found that adolescents who were exposed to online friends' display of risky behaviors such as smoking and drinking were significantly more at risk of following suit. The really interesting factor was that adolescents with actual face-to-face exposure of friends partaking in the same risky behaviors were less likely to follow suit.[160] My take on this again is regarding the learning of real-life boundaries that do not translate online. Online, a selfie of a kid posing with a bottle looks pretty cool, in real life drunk, perhaps less so. Offline or in face-to-face interaction, one is also exposed to the uncool aspects of adolescent exploration of alcohol: the talking too loud, the slurring and spitting with speech, getting overemotional, the fighting, and of course getting sick. In real life kids experience the altered state of alcohol and the perceived fun or adrenaline rush of deviance (that comes with underage drinking), but they also witness the downside; they see and smell the vomit. They stay real.

Children: The New Market

Last, but definitely not least, extracurricular arts and sports have increasingly become a capitalistic venture as opposed to a cultural or community pursuit. They cost money, big money! i-tech, even the latest and the greatest, is considerably more affordable.

Parents are spending massive amounts of money on activities that are constructed for profit under the guise of cultural broadening, education, or athleticism: for example, dance schools that compete against each other, routinely requiring costumes, travel, and parents to buy tickets to all the shows above and beyond the cost of the lessons. This is no longer about gaining grace, poise, athleticism, team spirit, or any of the other positives that an informal dance education usually provides. It is pure capitalistic venture. The schools are creating their own competition, their own market. And parents are buying in.

Same with some sport; parents pay extra to give a child the highest quality of professional equipment, to be able to play a specific position in hockey, or be placed in a certain number of competition games, or to have a specific coach. I have not even mentioned the role of the "correct" brand or label on children's equipment.

Forget jerseys and cleats, all you fundamentally need to play soccer is a ball. Same holds true of most sports; they can be enjoyed quite stripped down. Ice hockey becomes street ball (costing approximately twenty dollars for a cheap stick and a tennis ball as opposed to the hundreds, or for that matter thousands required for the skates, protective equipment, rink time, gas to drive to practice, etc.). Equally, tennis can be played against school walls, or in many communities at free courts. Whatever happened to kick the can? Why do children now *need* extensive and expensive equipment for play?

Unfortunately the "needs" for play are also being projected outwards; I am witnessing more and more parents and community collectively buying into the notion of children being perceived as underprivileged or uncared for when not provided with the best or the latest opportunity or equipment. No one is winning here except the providers of said exclusive equipment. We must re-differentiate between sport as play and generalized skill acquisition versus as training for elite professional positions. They are different and should not be confounded.

An interesting aside that may be noteworthy and give us all real food for thought: in a David Suzuki documentary,[161] on the great quest to find out why Olympians and other elite runners from specific regions of Africa were systematically, literally and figuratively beating all other athletes by miles, the most interesting fact was presented. It was not genetics, brain physiology, or body structure; many other athletes from other regions were blessed with drive and determination, the classic long lean legs and strong buttocks we see across our television screens or at athletic events. The winning advantage was being raised shoeless. Being raised working and walking barefoot on tough arduous farm land due to incredible poverty resulted in the most incredible feet. The strongest, toughest, springy and pliable, truly magnificent feet that could later allow a child to fly!

So before we spend oodles of money on our children, including campaigning and contributing to "poor" children's art and sport funds, I highly suggest we consider letting go of the notions of teams that involve substantial financial investment, organization, uniformity, uniforms, and, yes, driving. Bring back clubs, community clubs: give to a community center that subsidizes kids' art, music, language, and sport programs, or Big Brothers and Big Sisters, which foster relationships over events. Back to sport, if the children want to compete, they can by forming teams of the children present. If they don't, there is no obligation to play for other than for fun. If they really have emergent talent, the word will spread; a team, official club, or scout will find them (so too will a community or a sponsor).

A Walk Through History – How Did We Get Here?

The way a family unit functions has changed substantially over the past fifty years. Now that in most communities the nuclear family, and localized extended family, is the minority, parents often fend entirely on their own, employing day care, babysitters, after school programs, and sport and arts programs where financially viable or necessary. Parents are uncomfortable or feel they will be burdening a neighbor to mind a child for an hour or two when something comes up. Bottom line, there is no longer community reciprocity for child care. So we buy it.

We now also have less unstressed or non–objective-related parent-child time and family interaction in general: the concept of spending *quality* time as opposed to just being around with a child (or for that matter a partner) becomes an accepted if not a necessary concept to rationalize our otherwise extended absences from our children, friends, and partners. In the specific case of children, there is now a perceived need to entertain, explicitly teach, or occupy a child now that day-to-day inclusion has come into conflict with all that needs to be done, never mind parental need for personal time, couple time, or rest.

In recent years what I believe to be a guilt model has been emerging, thinly veiled in child-centered parenting. As just discussed, even when not needed for child care, parents spend immense amounts of time (and money) taxiing children to practices, tournaments, competitions, and lessons of all sorts, feeling like lesser or insufficient parents if they cannot provide these supplemental educational, sport, or artistic opportunities for their children. And yes, the play date: even the need for the scheduling of play. In parenting, we have shifted from an inclusion model to an accommodation model. And, when absolutely burdened or exhausted, an isolation model: we isolate our children with i-tech.

In recent years what I believe to be a guilt model has been emerging, thinly veiled in child-centered parenting.

When did all this start? In short, when children started to be in conflict as opposed to cohesion; when children started to conflict with work and industry; when the very notion of family itself conflicted with all one had to do.

Parental work patterns in combination with diminished support systems for young families have left parents in higher states of stress and fatigue. Children seem much, much more demanding in a system that no longer has the time to foster them. Many parents feel massively overworked, stressed, and downright too fatigued to play with, never mind be simply present with, their children. Something is upside down.

Now it is very easy to blame all this on working mothers. But the marginalization of parenting and family itself started long before this cultural trend. Keep in mind, apart from the biological imperative of human gestation (AKA pregnancy), birthing, and breastfeeding, the great majority of parenting can be fulfilled by either gender, and facilitated by all.

This marginalization of parenting undoubtedly is magnified by cultural attitude, what I see as a definitive anti-family or anti-parent tone in larger culture. We now mock or tease men for driving minivans and SUVs as opposed to sport cars. We criticize women for a post-pregnancy bump or loss of skin tone, for wearing "mom jeans" or otherwise accommodating the natural figure and lifestyle changes that come with parenting and parenthood. Men used to be admired for the virility that came with the trophy of children, and women were sought out for functional bodies conducive to childbirth and child rearing including curvy hips and real as opposed to silicone breasts. Now I'm not saying we should return to notions of antiquity (and the many accompanying negatives), but rather we should stop undermining parents, the jobs they do, and the choices and sacrifices they make, and try to shift back to a society that is family inclusive.

Family Inclusive

It was not always this way. Take the school year. It was specifically designed for family life in an agricultural society. Children were initially off in the summer not because it was too warm, or because it was cruel not to let them play outside, but because it was a burden to get them there. There was a cost to their formal education. The family was taxed with educational needs and requirements in conflict with family needs.

In late spring through summer to early fall, children were needed at home, the older to take care of the younger, and to tend to newborn animals and crops. This was the busy season in farming, and many hands, even the littlest of hands, were needed for tending, for harvesting, and later for preserving food for winter. In the early modernization of the world, children and their seasonal education were a part of the system, not in conflict with it. The educational system set in place was complementary. The system was adapted to the family and its needs. The family reigned.

We Have it Backwards

Now it is the opposite; culturally we have not adapted, at least not in a homeostatic way. Summer, or school vacation, for many families is an increased burden, including a financial burden. Parents must seek out and pay for camps, day care, or other services to care for their children while they remain on a standard work cycle. And, as will be explored shortly, they now also want their money's worth!

When it Got Messy

In the history of families, things started to get really messy with the expansion of industry, when more and more parents started to work for others instead of for or in their own proper family – when parents increasingly started to work in mines, factories, and larger offices or companies as opposed to their own shops, trades, or on their own farms.

In the not too distant past, and still in some traditional family businesses, when the schooling day was over, children joined their parents, partook and helped, or self-occupied. In restaurants, they prepped food, folded napkins, did their homework, or played at a back table as their parents worked. Now, in most jobs, parents have to go home at the end of the school day (rather than at the end of the work day) or they need to find and pay for alternate care for their children. The system is no longer in sync: financially or otherwise.

Since the late 1800s in England, industry is the reason why children were sent off to schooling earlier and earlier: to liberate parents, primarily women, to return them to the work force earlier. Not for the women's own benefit nor for their children, but for industry itself. Enter the need for day care under the guise of education. In Canada, day care, which later evolved into kindergarten, and a six dollar per month baby bonus, to pay for it, was introduced as part of the war effort in 1944. (Irony of the German name indeed, and darned good money in 1944). My point is, the system adapted rather quickly when women were needed for specific war duties or to take over at jobs men, now at war, had previously filled.

Now this is the really interesting factor: early education is not a good thing. It also halts development. Why? This is the time for play! Unstructured play is where learning at this age truly occurs.

Unstructured play is where learning at this age truly occurs.

Play Versus Learning: Educational Brainwashing

This factoid seems counterintuitive to us, the now modern brainwashed. Yet, it has been quite consistently found that starting formal schooling, e.g., your maths and your letters (literacy and numeracy) before age seven, is not only often not helpful, it can be damaging.[162] It is also a primary cause of much anxiety and many behavioral issues. Little one's brains have not been formally set up yet by other forms of pre-learning for systematic learning (they physically haven't had enough time on the planet yet for the brain to develop to such a state).

In support of this concept are some interesting early findings on learning disabilities, amongst them ADHD, that unfortunately did not get much attention. In the 1980s and early 1990s, when ADHD had it's first "surge," it was found that children born in spring and summer were the ones with the learning disabilities; in other words, children eight to twelve months younger than their classmates. There is no disability here, just eight to twelve months less development – cognitive, emotional, and kinetic development – due to the Fall cut-off age of entry for Kindergarten or Grade One. Of course these children were more challenged than their classmates. They were not stupid, uncoordinated, or inattentive; they were younger! In a sum total of five to six years, eight to twelve months is a big developmental gap: it's one fifth of a life!

This phenomenon, termed the relative age effect, was widely publicized in professional sport, specifically hockey (and yes, when speaking about young men: no longer children). Children born closer to cut-off dates have intellectual as well as physical or kinetic disadvantages when compared to their older peers. Older children have a greater advantage; they are physically as well as cognitively more prepared for learning and hence better performance.[163] For whatever reason, however, this effect was largely ignored in education and the notion of educational disabilities took over.[164]

Back to Play-Based Learning

But we can't turn back the clock to pre-industry, pre-war, or pre–single parenthood, nor should we. Culture is progressing and child care is needed for most single or dual parent families regardless.

Quite early on, a few philosophers, psychologists, and educators were in tune with the educational or developmental purpose(s) of play and attempted to bridge multiple societal needs (and misconceptions). Enter play-based learning. Play-based learning philosophies or schools, the most famous of them Montessori, sought to fulfill children's social and learning needs with the side benefit of fulfilling societal needs. Play-based learning programs provided a place to put children while parents were working and served the dual purpose of acclimating them to future schooling. They were really on to something good: a most welcomed alternative to the ruler and fear used in the past to get little ones to sit still and absorb and to methylphenidate today (now that corporal punishment and teacher bullying are no longer accepted practice to ensure children's attention and behavioral compliance to their lessons).

Unfortunately there is, and has been, far too much room for misinterpretation and hence mis-application of the expert knowledge of these brilliant early childhood educators. I can't tell you how many educational disasters I have seen from otherwise well-educated and well-intentioned parents who teach their children absolutely nothing before sending them to school. Equally calamitous are the train wrecks from children who emerge from supposed Montessori and other similar schools who have had their learning restricted under the guise of the otherwise brilliant concept of play-based learning.

Not formal does not mean none, stalling, or delaying interest; it also does not mean i-tech. It means play and exposure, including reading to your child daily at home, having them gain curiosity for letters and numbers and their collective meaning(s). A great American philosopher, Paul Goodman, spoke of a utopian world wherein learning to read and write could, would, and should be by osmosis. Indeed the concept makes a lot of sense – presuming parents are well educated themselves and they have, and take, the time to mentor and coach their children through various learning processes, including the learning of words and letters. I don't know about you, but when I look around me, most parents are starved themselves for such time, leaving most, if not all of their children's learning, in the hands of formal educators.

...when I look around me, most parents are starved themselves for such time...

The great and sad irony here is that the evolutionary and true purpose of play itself is learning: cognitive and emotional learning. The whole concept of replacing play with learning in early childhood is entirely oxymoronic.

There is also mounting evidence that formal learning too young promotes anxiety, and that other mental health issues are seeded in performance requirements of (far too) early formal schooling. This is precisely the time for play. From zero to six, and many would even say seven, children learn almost exclusively through play. Of note, countries that start formal education later, namely Sweden, Finland, and Denmark, as opposed to England, the US, and Canada, have some of the highest comparative literacy rates and highest level of general education in the general populace.

You probably also noted my sarcasm a few paragraphs back regarding methylphenidate or other medications being used to control children in classrooms. What does this tell us? Why did we need to use fear and hurt children in the past or medicate them in the present to ensure their attention and behavioral compliance to learning? Today's widespread practice of using pharmaceuticals for schooling needs to be examined. Perhaps children are not ready. Perhaps they are just behaving like children. Perhaps there is nothing wrong with children at all: past or present. Perhaps there is something wrong with our expectations of them, of ourselves.

So What is Play? And Why Not i-Play?

The True Purpose of Play

Play serves many purposes: social learning, environmental learning, conceptual development, and state regulation, all of which can be thwarted when the role is given exclusively to digital media. The key here again is to remember that with the very young, unlike other toys and games, digital media risks replacing or re-directing natural developmental process.

While playing on i-tech does fulfil or perhaps I should say

mimic learning process(es), it also, by its very nature, supersedes some of the developmental processes playing is designed to engage: primarily again in social learning, environmental learning, emotional learning, and its cohort state regulation or emotional regulation governed by the nervous system.

Most i-games promote the development of strategy, including spatial planning and working memory through identification, recognition, and the moving of things, which are arguably not so important in the early phases of development. In fact, what research has also routinely shown us is, especially in early childhood, the less structured the play, the better. Again by the very design of the mechanism or technology, this is reversely limited; the processes in i-tech are by definition completely structured – they are programmed.

In fact, what research has also routinely shown us is, especially in early childhood, the less structured the play, the better.

What Children Naturally Explore

Watch young children on a field with a ball, with no adults around. No adult directing, mitigating, or refereeing. Children will not play by official rules; they negotiate. In fact they get rather irritated by the little guy reminding them all the time of "the rules." Leaders and followers appear. Rules will alter for inclusion as well as exclusion. It is equally likely that a group of children will make a new rule to exclude a child disliked or in bullying for sport (experimenting with power and control, the negatives of leadership per se) as it is they will alter a rule for inclusion, narrow goal posts, shorten the field, or not obstruct a pass so that a weaker or smaller child will experience victory.

True learning is experimental learning. It is organic. Seeing what will happen if...and what will happen when...how it feels if...and how it feels when.... It is the learning of boundaries such as weight, strength, and pliability of objects and materials, the exploration of the limitations of rules, of emotions, of relationships, even of physical pain, of power, or matter, of color, of distance, of anything, absolutely anything in our physical, emotional, spiritual, and fantasy world(s).

True or unbound learning is not learning what a game itself will or will not do, or will or will not allow one to do based on its programmed boundaries. The latter is limited learning. It is the form of learning we apply when we need or want to learn how to use a tool. Don't get me wrong: this form of learning definitely has its place, and a very important one at that, but that place should not be universal. Besides, children will get much of this formal or structured learning later in their education, in the higher grades.

Unstructured Play: Children Left to Their Own Devices

Now all that said, observing children, one will find unstructured play has its own little formula. When I observe children I find the majority of unguided play involves three components, with their order and relative weight shifting rather consistently. First, all play tends to involve some form of observation followed in no particular order by experimentation and problem solving, substitution, and social mimicry. Children will see or find objects and examine them, observe color, shape, form, texture, etc. (and yes, at certain stages, taste). They will then often experiment on how they may fit or function together or apart, roll them, tap them, throw them, layer them, etc. They will then pretend, or make believe they are other things. Lastly they will play with how they socially intermingle. Take any object(s), say some sticks and a leaf or two. A child will observe and trace the patterns in a leaf, perhaps notice it leaves a green film on their fingers and then scrape it on the pavement drawing or making "green paint," perhaps then poke around with the stick, pierce a leaf with the stick, or poke some ants with it. They then might construct something with the two components and start to make believe the stick and leaf combo they made can fly (pretend they are insects or perhaps a plane, spaceship, or whatever other item their little brain comes up with). They will then have them engage. This can be pro-social as in flying together, making patterns, or anti-social such as fighting each other: both equally valid explorations. When through, they then might start building a stick wall in front of the ants, disturb them and even squash some to observe what the ants will do. And finally perhaps they will devise an ant bridge with the leaf over the sticks to help the critters back on their route.

This play cycle, and in fact all non-digital (or otherwise non-computerized or non-programmed play), involves observation and a void space from which children come up with their own ideas: creative ones as well as conceptual ones. Children observe true structure and function, explore and invent structure and function, and thereafter create and solve problems (social, emotional, functional, structural, etc.) through play. They explore reality and fantasy, the abstract and the concrete, function and meaning.

Of note, social mimicking in play will follow what children observe and how they feel. For example, when playing dolls or house, children will mimic what they see in their proper families. They will also explore their emotions. An otherwise mentally healthy girl who is mad at her mother, for whatever reason, will make the mother character (or any character for that matter) particularly evil toward the child or other character for an afternoon or a week or however long she needs to process her emotions toward her mother and their relationship. Although perhaps disconcerting for a parent to overhear, most children also resolve the issue through this play: that is the explicit purpose of the process. Mommy and baby doll, as well as friend dolls, will eventually explore making up, just as they do, or wish, in real life.

Social mimicking will also follow the rules provided, meaning if children watch programs and then are given character dolls and toys as opposed to abstract dolls, they will role play in character with less creative freedom. For example Barbie will act like Barbie,

My Little Pony will follow the story line as observed on TV, as will Spider Man, SpongeBob SquarePants, and Transformer. If you wish your children to be more creative or not mimic that which they see on media, leave the void, give them abstract as opposed to character toys.

So Why Do We Want It?

So if all this unstructured imaginative play is so good for kids, why do they, or for that matter, *we* crave i-media?

Here is where all the science, theories, and cultural trends merge. First, little kids don't crave i-media by nature any more than any other toy, game, or device; they start to desire it for all the social-developmental reasons outlined above. And then, just like adults, they get caught in the structure, the pull, of the medium itself, unfortunately with potentially wider reaching (developmental) consequences. Second, kids naturally mimic. They mimic their parents and elders, their siblings and peers. If we are playing on our tablets, texting away on our phones and working on computers, they want to as well. It will become part of their play and then their reality. Last, by introducing the medium far too early we train little brains to need entertainment as opposed to seeking it or making it themselves. We remove the critical first step, observation, followed by the second, curiosity. Many of us (not just scholars, educators, and health care providers including MDs, psychologists and psychiatrists; the general populace too) are concerned with the effects of over-programming or otherwise over-organization of children's time (including play time) on learning and intelligence.

Let me leave you with some thoughts from art and popular culture. A few lines delivered by a character in the film *Late Bloomers* summed things up beautifully: "I want you to be bored; it's good for the imagination" and later "people who don't know how to be bored grow up to be idiots."[165]

CHAPTER TEN

Socialization Part A: Child's Play

In the last two chapters I looked at how i-tech had found its niche as an electronic babysitter in the post-modern family. I examined the purpose of play, learning, and attachment in the larger developmental picture including i-tech's role in potentially thwarting critical phases of developmental process in infants and children.

In this chapter, I will start a discussion on how in the name of discipline, safety, and humaneness, i-tech has found yet another niche. How, for better or for worse, i-tech is now the principal tool of relational exploration and the primary modality of boundary exploration for children, adolescents, and youth.

Starting with the story of the demise of the play fight and other forms of aggressive mimicking, I will examine how restriction in non-digital forms of physical play may actually be associated with an increase in true aggressive expression on- and offline. In this context, I will explore the role each may have in the lack of learning of true physical and emotional boundaries in the "real world." I will speak directly to bullying, its secret sister relational aggression, and the special

> ...for better or for worse, i-tech is now the principal tool of relational exploration and the primary modality of boundary exploration for children, adolescents, and youth.

role i-tech plays in the reduction of inhibitions and the magnification of negative affect.

Play: Fighting, Comradery, and Romance

In all mammals, including us, play fighting is a primary means of making and thereafter maintaining social bonds. It is a way of testing new relationships, establishing trust, and negotiating inclusion and one's role in social hierarchy. In warring tribes or nations it is also training for combat. For young boys in particular, the testing of trust is key in gaining affiliation; it is a means to integrate into groups. Will your new friend or opponent actually go too far and hurt you, or will he stop with play? What will he do when he has the upper hand? How does he act when you have the upper hand? Does he cry, squeal, laugh, yell, run to Mommy or the teacher, bring on Dad or a big brother, negotiate, wait for revenge? Is he overt or is he sneaky; does he use brains or brawn? How does he repair the situation when things do go too far? All of these very social questions are asked, answered, and negotiated though play, commonly through play fighting or what we used to call roughhousing.[166]

As we get older gentle aggressive play does not necessarily dissipate. It is still a common tool of social exploration: a way to test the waters per se. For example, gentle aggression is commonly used to explore potential for romance in otherwise established relationships such as platonic friendships. Watching adolescents and many adults, you will note they will gently tap or bump; adolescents and youth will even tumble, say in tickling fights, as a way of testing boundaries prior to caressing, the unquestionable romantic advance.[167] Adult males and some females also continue to lightly tap, push, bump hips, and fake punch playfully with their closer friends as a means of maintaining closeness or again when (re) negotiating affiliation in groups. We need this form of physical interplay. It has social-developmental and biological purpose.

Exploratory Aggression, No Place for It, No Way, No Where

In North America, somewhere along the line, we lost our perspective on what we used to refer to as child's play. Just as with the restrictions we now place on "dangerous" objects or toys in playgrounds like ladders, teeter-totters, and high swings, so too in interpersonal play we are focusing on the potential for harm, as opposed to physical socio-emotional learning (and fun). We appear to have lost our ability to differentiate between the healthy learning of social and physical boundaries in play and the expression of overt aggression with intent to harm. Just as kids get scratches and bumps and occasionally truly hurt falling off bikes, monkey bars, or swings, so too they can occasionally get hurt in the play fight. It is part of the social and physical learning the activity is designed to evoke. Such play indeed evokes the need for the true learning of boundaries.

I fear we have lost sight of this natural interplay; our focus is now rather exclusively one sided, on the negatives of rough play. We now focus on bullying, true aggression often veiled in play, as opposed to the occasional price of the accidental or exploratory bump.

> There is no platform for positive (as well as negative) boundary exploration under the sharp eyes of elders.

This attitude shift has left us with zero tolerance policies for all unorganized aggressive or physical play.[168] The unexpected fallout, however, is that this blanket restriction leaves children with no outlet for interpersonal physicality. There is no platform for positive (as well as negative) boundary exploration under the sharp eyes of elders. The point blank restriction format may also be contributing to the current increase in intensity of bullying when it does occur. I also believe it is responsible for an increase in covert aggression.

So where does i-tech fit in? Quite simply, it is the substitute for play fighting, the new delivery system for relational aggression, and thereafter the emotional processing system, or rather, the emotional "non-processing" system.

In the socialization process, when we remove something that serves emotional, developmental or relational purpose, something else (positive or negative) will inevitably fill the perceived need or actual void. In the case of aggressive mimicking and frustration, they cannot simply be repressed. All behaviors and emotions (good and bad) need exploratory, as well as defusing, venues including effective processing time. Children, and adults for that matter, need processes that foster relationship building and social bonding. We are wired this way. If we suppress or do not provide access to one method, another will find its place. This is indeed the case with gaming. Where roughhousing and play fighting used to be the tool of social bonding, now gaming is.

The New Play

Early gaming did not include the testing of social boundaries, the testing and learning of limits of play and pain (e.g., physical and emotional hurt), nor did it really explore the testing of loyalty. Today, computer games have evolved considerably and many games do include many, if not all, of the above features. Hence, we should not be surprised that they have become the primary tool of social bonding for many children, adolescents, and youth.

A couple of studies have found that children who game up to one hour a day are quite psychosocially adjusted.[169] Now for the fine print. As outlined in previous chapters, we must be very cautious of globalizing or generalizing the positives and negatives of research. We also must be careful of our omissions. From my professional perspective, emphasis should be not on the game–no game debate, but on the duration and context of gaming when it does occur. The theme repeated *ad nauseum* in this book is "nothing wrong with a little, a lot wrong with a lot." The second theme is integration versus interference. In keeping with the parameters of these two themes, if gaming is integrated in play and friendships, this can be perfectly healthy and indeed a lot of fun. If it completely replaces face-to-face relationships or other forms of play, it most definitely is not.

When we examine who is socially adjusted and who is not, it is not just about the gaming; it is also about the surrounding family dynamic, attachment and peer circles or lack thereof, and individual neurological liability. Two boys from healthy families, who also ride their bikes, bug their sisters, and play soccer or baseball together are probably well-adjusted children who also happen to enjoy gaming together. Two boys who have never met in person, who play MMOs for hours on end as teammates in fantasy roles, who have no other interests, no offline friends, and get very upset at each other or their parents when they are unable to play at the expected times are invariably not.

All this said, there is a lot of gray in the middle. As discussed in earlier chapters, gaming is directly associated with elevated instances of learning disorders and compromised socialization abilities. Repeating the rule of thumb: no more than one hour of screen time a day for older children, absolutely none until the age of four; and waiting until six is notably healthier. There is far too much socialization, emotional regulation, heck everything, being learned and hardwired in the very young years, and kids under six are absolute sponges; you want them to relate to you and absorb what you teach, not that which i-tech and media do.

There is far too much socialization, emotional regulation, heck everything, being learned and hardwired in the very young years, and kids under six are absolute sponges; you want them to relate to you and absorb what you teach, not that which i-tech and media do.

The New Fight

A theme you might notice building through the last few chapters is that of boundaries: how and where we learn them and subsequently how and where we apply them, or not. As the name of the activity itself denotes, the play fight is a social learning activity that not only is a physical outlet but also directly explores the social boundaries of play and fighting: the rules of socio-emotional interaction.

i-tech gaming is a social activity that does some of this but always within the limits of a specific program; besides, it is not really you, it is a character (or an object) you are operating in a constructed reality. So what or where is the new outlet? Where can children explore emotions and the boundaries of physicality, aggression, and the limits of each? How or through what do they find out what truly hurts? And what is the price of limiting such exploratory process?

New Tools and Old Methods

For young girls, historically, cultural intolerance of physical aggression, anger, and negative sentiment in general resulted in covert relational aggression or what we now refer to as the Mean Girl phenomenon. This form of aggression is anything but new, but it is now magnified. With i-tech as the new operational tool, we are seeing more and more of it.

Relational aggression, once typically associated with repressed or otherwise forbidden "unladylike" emotions in females, is now increasingly common in boys. This emotional-behavioral gender crossing, I believe, has two catalysts. It is in part due to the new delivery tool, i-tech, but also directly related to the suppression of physical play. When we suppress physical play or physical expression, boys, just like girls, will find other means of expressing themselves, and these means are not necessarily better.

When we suppress physical play or physical expression, boys, just like girls, will find other means of expressing themselves, and these means are not necessarily better.

There is some historical-cultural support for this. Think of cultures or communities of men which restrict physicality for conflict resolution, e.g., educational or religious communities. Under such political conditions men, just like women, essentially use brains over brawn to not only resolve conflict but also to cause it. Spousal jokes aside, the fundamental difference between men and boys is men are socially and emotionally developed human beings; they are wielding tools fully knowing and wanting a specific desired (negative or positive) outcome. Boys in contrast, purely by function of their years on the planet, are not fully developed socially or otherwise. By nature of their limited years, boys are often unaware of much of the true potential impact of their actions; they are still learning.

I believe it may be time for us to very seriously re-examine our stance on attitudes toward, and definitions of, aggression in children. For all, and surely evident with girls, covert aggression can be far more damaging than the overt expression of the original (suppressed) anger.[170] Covert aggression is further significantly harder to identify and manage effectively due to its insidious nature. It thus spirals out of hand (including out of parental or authority's control) much more easily. As will be discussed in detail shortly hereafter, it also becomes grossly and often tragically magnified with i-tech; more and more children are now committing suicide over it.

The time may have come to re-examine the relative weight of occasional physical versus systematic emotional scarring and how we choose to intervene with each. Attempts to mitigate violence in the school(yard) by pacifying or feminizing young males with zero tolerance for aggressive play as well as efforts to repress females' expression of frustration and anger appear to be leading to a heightened desire for relational aggression. It may also be related to an increased desire for other aggressive experience in general, for example, bashing someone's head in with a baseball bat in Grand Theft Auto.[171]

Unfortunately, in our current socio-political environment, parents, guardians, and educators who dismiss aggressive behavior or aggressive mimicking as a natural part of childhood are now perceived as part of the problem.[172] We are viewed as morally unsophisticated or at best inattentive to the (ac)culturation of children. This dismissed counterposition, and the one I tend to hold to professionally, however, is based upon much more than the age-old *laissez faire* adage of "let boys be boys," or "let the girls run wild." It is based upon the principle that absolute non-tolerance of aggressive play (aggressive mimicking), and negative sentiment, leads to children and youth being attracted to accessible mediums that allow for the exploration or expression of such sentiment. They now look for it.

And they find it. Covertly and overtly, they find it relationally through social media (Facebook, texting, etc.) or through violent gaming. And, at least relationally, the true aggression is much, much, more intense and unbridled when it does occur. It is also not monitored.

The Kids Need Us!

Neufeld and Maté[173] also believe that bullying and child and youth aggression are misunderstood. They too believe that they are based in frustration, but equally important, in the eroding of generational hierarchy. The point I am adding is that extreme bullying may also be due to the loss of healthy venues for the expression of natural physicality, and the ability to (healthily) defuse true anger. I perceive mean girls to be frustrated girls who take out their frustration relationally because they do not see or know of any other "acceptable" venue for the healthy expression of anger (or said frustration). It is now much the same for boys.

In the great debate of whether violent media and gaming is the cause or a principal contributor to extreme bullying, Neufeld and Maté again adhere to their perspective that extreme acts of aggression and bullying of children and adolescents are rooted in peer orientation due to the loss of attachment hierarchy with parents. They find peer attachment, as opposed to parental attachment, is conducive to increased exploration of dominance and submissiveness with said peers.

In certain phases of development, kids today, like kids of old, often want to be and often are left to their own devices, rather than those of, or taught by, their elders. Which, again, is fine with healthy attachment as, when out of their depth, they will return to elders for advice and such. But what happens when they don't look to us?

This leads us full circle back to the discussion in the chapter on attachment. Without attachment to a parent, parent or adult opinion is not valued or sought, nor is it consciously or instinctually followed. Even when it is given, many children (and youth) today are simply no longer responsive to parental direction. It does not hold value within their peer system.[174]

In sum, without parental attachment, parents and adults are no longer in charge of the behavioral management or development of their child(ren), leaving the natural dominant-passive relationship of caregivers and parents to children absent. As such, children and youth are now seeking out other relationships wherein the rules of dominant and passive are not clear. The instinct to dominate other children (and youth) arises when youth look to their equally socially and developmentally immature peers as opposed to responsible and mature adults for models of how to behave.[175]

The danger in this peer orientation model of bullying is not only that it can spiral out of control with greater speed, but that the bullies are no longer social outcasts as was common in the past. In peer orientation models, bullies are admired for their dominance, as parents and adults in general once were. Peer orientation also makes bullying far more dangerous as bullies are now not only feared, they are revered, and thus rewarded for their aggression with followings.[176] When this flip happens, the bullying also ceases to be covert: it becomes public on platforms accessed by peers (and usually only peers). Parents and elders are excluded (unless, that is, parents, teachers, and elders in general choose to govern social behaviors on their children's social media and phones).

In phases of development wherein it is natural to want to explore pushing boundaries (e.g., adolescence), kids may not want us, but they sure as heck need us. Just as with little children, they still need us to occasionally yet systematically check in, intervene, and (re)direct when necessary. Which brings us to a compounding factor of i-tech: in states of anger and frustration, i-tech is not only functioning as a tool of communication, it is functioning as a tool of emotional processing.

Emotional Processing

As discussed in the first chapters, we are no longer taking time to process. We are no longer allowing ourselves to sit in blank spaces to think, contemplate, and reflect. Neither are children, and in times where it would be most important to do so.

Post–corporal punishment and pre–i-tech, when children and adolescents "did wrong," pretty common interventional practice was to give them processing time. We told them to go to their rooms, or think about what they had done or were going to do. When things got extreme, we grounded the older ones and gave the little ones a time-out. But kids are not taking "time-out" figuratively or otherwise (past the formalized three minutes or so we actually give them). They are not processing independently. Unless otherwise restricted, once reprimanded, they are turning directly to their i-devices and games.

Children and adolescents now defuse through aggression or dissemination of information on i-tech. Awaiting empathy or reaction, they vent publicly or in pseudo-fantasy as opposed to effectively processing emotions in reality and relative quiet. They spontaneously post, they text, they game. They do not think. The problem here is when children and youth are truly angry and truly frustrated, this anger is not dissipated or defused by broadcasting via social media or with violent game play; in fact it increases with it, it fuels it, it gives it legs. In my view, this explains the connection between verbal aggression, violent game play, violent behavior, and bullying in the real world: again not for all, but surely for many.

Parents, and educators by proxy, may now be caught in yet another proverbial catch-22. By thwarting attachment, media and i-tech exposure may be a root cause, or key contributor to increased aggression in children and adolescents that parents and society try to mitigate by zero tolerance policies. Media and gaming industries are, however, completely in tune with the needs for such expression and use this (forbidden) desire to market products that allow children to vent out restricted attitudes and behavior(s). They got us.

As a clinician witnessing many otherwise lovely and intelligent children explore very negative and extremely harmful behaviors, I ask parents, educators, caregivers, and policy makers to re-examine what constitutes what we used to refer to as roughhousing (aggressive mimicking) and the expression of frustration versus overt aggression. I recommend that we draw the line with overt or covert intent to hurt. And perhaps most important of all, that we, the elders, do not leave the job of teaching what hurts, emotionally, physically, or relationally, to educational games or programs, media or other outside industry: that we take back the job ourselves from day one.

But there is more fueling all this. It is not just the means by which children (and elders for that matter) are defusing, it is also the method: the method and its effect on accompanying behavior.

Introducing the Disinhibition Effect – Expression in the Digital Age

There is just something about the digital screen that makes some of us act a little different. We are a little more out there, more brazen. We flirt; we share things we would think twice about sharing face to face. There is also something about the screen that makes *some* of us act *a lot* different. We bully, we troll, audaciously sext, and are otherwise more aggressive in our communication. So what is it? What is the medium doing to our personal communication "settings," to our communication style?

Cyberbullying

With children, the first area in which we notice rather dramatic change is again bullying: enter cyberbullying. Bullying has always been an issue. Not to dismiss it, but it has always been around. It is one of the unfortunate negatives of human nature. That said, bullying of yesteryear cannot approach what bullying can today. Cyberbullying has a reach and resulting power that bullying in the past did not. I have already discussed the role of repression and peer orientation; now I would like to address the role of i-tech itself. But first, what is bullying?

So what is bullying and why is it so powerful? Bullying usually takes two forms: one-on-one and group. In one-on-one bullying, one child (or adult) selects a victim and proceeds to make his or her life a living hell. One-on-one bullying can take multiple forms: actual violence, physical threat and emotional torture, as well as attack on property. Individuals cause physical or emotional pain through actions and words meant to attack one's sense of self, self-esteem or self-value, or sense of safety, or devalue or destroy what is dear to us. The formula is simple and the perpetrator thereafter thrives on the pain and fear of the victim and the resulting unequal power dynamic.

Bullying can also involve community or peers. This is usually a process of "othering," involving one child or adolescent taking the lead and a troop joining in. The formula here is a group ostracizing based on perceived or created difference. In my childhood it was the nerd, the redhead, the fat kid, the small kid, or the kid of color. Now it's the gay kid, the shy kid, the unfashionable kid, the slut. The difference is irrelevant and may not even be real. What matters is that the troop buys in to the "difference" and the victim shows hurt. Again the group and its leader thrive off sucking the energy of the victim. Bullies and the entourage, like a virus, become more and more powerful the more they weaken the target.

As discussed above, bullying took a new twist a few years back with the instigation of zero tolerance policies for perceived physical violence in public schools. It also took a jump with social inclusion policies wherein teachers, school counselors, and other school staff would try to work to integrate loner kids into established social circles. An unexpected side effect of these policies was an increase in relational as opposed to physical bullying. You can guide people, including children, to be kind to each other but you cannot force or impose relationships. Kids don't like being told who to be friends with! None of us do...and we abreact, we act out accordingly.

Until the advent of social media, relational bullying was usually typical of female rather than male behavior, but no longer. It is a unisex "sport." It is also exceptionally powerful. This form of bullying also involves ostracizing but it has an insidious power as it is rarely provable. As it involves "forbidden" behavior and "forbidden" sentiment we are supposed to be above, it is explicitly designed to fly under the radar of authority (e.g., parents, coaches, and educators). As such, it tends to be very subtle, applying exclusion through a turn of phrase or intonation rather than explicit insult, degradation, or any observable behavior.[177] Not only is the victim initially not quite sure what is happening, caregivers (e.g., parents and teachers), precisely as intended, are commonly blind to it. The group gradually emotionally destabilizes the victim, who ironically, is often part of the social circle. Worse, perhaps, the perpetrators(s) are often themselves perceived as "good" kids with good grades. To external eyes the victim is part of the social group, included in most activities. Outsiders (AKA adults) can't perceive what is wrong.

Digital media has taken relational bullying to new heights leading to the extreme mass bullying that we now know can push a fragile teen or youth to suicide. Think mean girls on steroids. A key factor in its "success" is both the mass reach of digital media and the disinhibition effect. The combination means that there is truly no escape for the victim.

Mass Reach: Anytime, Everywhere, Everyone

The obvious is that social networks such as MySpace in the past and Facebook today have a very long arm: these networks reach a mass amount of people, instantly. You don't have to be walking past a bully or be at school to be affected. You can be reached and hurt anywhere, anytime, and everyone instantly knows it. The damage done by gossip in the cafeteria, over traditional land lines, at sleepovers, and in locker rooms of yesteryear was considerably slower. It took longer to create a rumor mill and longer for people to react or join in.

The impact, albeit terrible, was lesser. Bullying in the past was also situational; it occasionally stopped or paused. This is not a minor point. In the past, the bullied could usually find refuge, for example at home or in a different social circle. Today they cannot. There is no space digital media cannot reach, and there is no let-up.

In the past, the bullied could usually find refuge, for example at home or in a different social circle. Today they cannot.

The consistency and the speed of the bullying by social media, including texting and forwarding, is relentless, feeding upon itself even if the bullied do not respond. There is no escape. Instant messages are, well...instant. And when someone lets up, someone else picks up the torch and continues the process. All of this has an emotional compounding effect on the victim. The perception is that everyone is part of the bullying actively (or passively) all the time. It is a constant bombardment, a hailstorm of insult and injury.

How Did It Become So Extreme?

The Disinhibition Effect

In cyberbullying, lack of inhibition has taken over where peer pressure left off; and the compounding effect is monumental. Generally speaking, peer pressure makes us "forget" our own morals or belief structures when the need to belong is stronger. A person will sacrifice larger social judgment, hurting or participating in the bullying of another (child or adult), to not be alone, or to heighten their own social status by being included in the powerful as opposed to the weaker group. Peer pressure lowers inhibition, period.

Disinhibition is a little different. The term was coined by Cooper, Delmonico, and Burg[178] when explaining the cybersex phenomenon. Simply put, individuals engage in behavior they otherwise would not, not because of the protection provided by the mass as with peer pressure, but because of the perceived protection, and often the anonymity, provided by the screen. A third factor is that online rules are inherently different. Although times are changing, most often, repercussions for public or pseudo-public online behavior are minimal when compared to public offline behavior. Children and adolescents would be reprimanded, sent to the principal's office, a counselor or even expelled if they systematically lined up and yelled profanities, racial slurs, or the like at a passing child. Frequently nothing happens when all of the same are done (and deleted or streams removed) via i-tech.

Patterns and Roles in Cyberbullying

In cyberbullying, individuals tend to initiate, to test, fully protected behind the digital screen or within a designated online "friend" or peer circle. When there is no repercussion, or there is social reward by virtue of a following, they continue. Here, both peer pressure and disinhibition are in full effect, creating the perfect storm for social aggression. In cyberbullying, there are further additional dimensions to the traditional poles of aggressor and bystander.

In cyberbullying, individuals can partake in the bullying at any level: anonymous sheltered behind digital screens, overt with name and face attached, or as voyeur. They can also play double roles, which is a game that is viciously destabilizing to the intended victim (e.g., being very aggressive digitally and very pleasant or neutral in person). The irony is that no one is excluded in the process, including the individual being bullied. The overt, the covert, and the bystander all contribute to the downfall of the victim. Everyone is involved!

Feeding on the Worst of Human Nature

Aside from the obvious analogy to the euphoric psychodynamics of a feeding frenzy, other behavioral factors contribute to the phenomenon. Apart from peer orientation and disinhibition, some very scary or inhumane features of supposed humanity are here in full play:

1. The first is a play of numbers. Bottom line is if you are to be attacked, you want to be attacked with few people around. Sounds counterintuitive, but social psychology has proven this over and over again. If there are few people or only one person around when something unfortunate happens, an individual will usually react, take social responsibility, and come to your rescue. The feeling of social responsibility is stronger the smaller the group. The more people, the more people will assume someone else will, or should, help, and they will just walk on by. I believe the same social psychology rule is in effect with cyberbullying.

2. The second is the belief that participating only a little bit or as voyeur has no effect. All of us in these situations tend to be blind to the compounding effect. There are numerous analogies that apply. Take water in winter: one person may throw a cold bucket of water on a person's head, but it is the 100 people thereafter who drop only one drop, or do not take the individual in from the cold that will eventually lead to the person dying of hypothermia.

3. Lastly, the medium facilitates an altering or magnification of persona: meaning beyond disinhibition we act differently with i-tech (positive and negative). The altering of persona

by role, circumstance, or rules of engagement, however, is not a new human phenomenon. Once again, my running theme is that we cannot blame it all on i-tech. An example that is valid through the centuries is the military. In the military, putting on a uniform results in an individual conforming and performing the common duty. However, in the name of this common duty, the exact same uniform can transform one individual into a hero and another into a tyrant. The same holds true of the digital screen; behind it some of us abuse our newfound power and act like entirely different people.

What Can We Do?

Be There and Aware

All these very human features combine with i-tech to give cyber-bullying its full effect. So what can we do? I think the first step is to acknowledge how imperfect we are: that good people, never mind good kids, explore bad behavior too. I'm not saying to empathize with the bullies or have tolerance for those who assist them, but rather to open our eyes, stay closer to our children, and be there to guide when kids' games start to go bad. Maté and Neufeld's theory on the loss of attachment hierarchy again applies fully here. Children now turn to peers as opposed to elders to define their behavior. They model each other's impulsive actions rather than adults' conscientious thought. If, as a culture, we want to reduce the power and effect of cyberbullying, this trend needs to be reversed. Get closer to your kids. Control the digital devices you provide and purchase for them. Monitor their texting, email, and Facebook accounts and let them know you are doing so. This is not invasion of privacy; this is parenting!

The problem is not the exploration of nasty behavior per se; it is a natural phase for many adolescents (and two-year-olds). The problem is that the behavior snowballs unchecked. If the medium being used is not monitored by the older and wiser, or by those with the power to make it stop, quite simply, it won't. Parents, teachers, community leaders, and caretakers too frequently are unaware of it, or mis-measure the severity of it, until it is far too late. This is coupled with a new parental insecurity on boundaries of invading children's privacy.

As a community I believe we need to revive the parenting philosophy that privacy comes second to safety: safety from the less innocent, such as adult predators, but also from the naïve, other adolescents, and yes little children too, who get high on the power without realizing the devastation they cause. Cyberbullying is in essence the blind leading the blind, in games involving tools that now can kill.

Back to the medium itself, a key question is: Would we do it anyway? In the case of bullying, unfortunately, the answer is yes. We cannot and should not blame it all on i-tech. Texting and Facebook did not create nor cause bullying. They just represent a frighteningly efficacious medium that engages disinhibition, thwarts processing, and as such succeeds in engaging the worst rather than the best of human nature: hence the extreme harm potential.

CHAPTER ELEVEN

Socialization Part B: Adult Play (Sex & Sexuality)

Sex and the Net: Desensitization, Disinhibition, Arousal Templates, and the Death of Intimacy

And now, the chapter on sex. In no other area are we being so profoundly affected by i-tech as in the realm of sexuality. This should come as no surprise. It just makes sense: any medium or method that is blanketly affecting attachment, pair bonding, emotional regulation, availability, attention, communication, the learning of physical and emotional boundaries, inhibition, peer versus parental orientation, and yes anticipatory and arousal cycles (essentially everything discussed up to this point) is bound to affect sexuality. And has it ever!

My professional opinion on sexuality and sexual boundaries has to date been fairly liberal. Meaning, if adults and youth of age legally and knowingly consent, and there does not appear to be any deceit, abuse, or manipulation, who are we (those not directly involved in the relationship) to judge and pontificate what is right and wrong, healthy or unhealthy? My view is narrowing.

I am not so concerned about what Cooper, Delmonaco, and Burg[179] refer to as recreational sexual use of i-media, including the exploration or the broadening of sexual horizons and sexual fantasies some individuals explore on the Internet. Other mediums do the same. Case in point, the book *Fifty Shades of Grey*, like the *Story of O* long before it, gave a little jump to many bedrooms. The sensational success of the series also implies that many people wanted such a jump. What I am concerned about is the adjunct acceleration and broadening of sexual expectations, resulting in individuals consenting to things they are uncomfortable with, not because they are curious or want to explore them, but because they feel they no longer have a choice.

Is the "New Normal" the "Internet Normal"?

What I am concerned about are the changes in our attitudes and our desires that go far beyond the frameworks of curiosity and a bit of fun. The central issue once again concerns "moreness." The endless availability, variety, and novelty of sexual content as provided on the Internet has taken the sexual game higher. The questions we are now left with are: Do we all want to play by Internet rules? And do we remain healthy in games with such high stakes?

Do we all want to play by Internet rules? And do we remain healthy in games with such high stakes?

But first, who made the new rules?

The Porn Industry

Via the Internet, the porn industry gained a reach like it never had before. And, as a capitalistic business, much like the beauty industry before it, it gradually redefined our notions of sex and sexuality through the propagation of imagery.

Sexual Beauty

Porn on the net has globally affected our sexual behavior, all of our sexual behavior. It is redefining sexual desirability as well as sexual beauty. Through acting and images it is telling us what we should do, and what we should look like to be desirable mates; in sum, it is telling us we should look and act like those on our screens. And we are listening. In this redefining via sexual imagery, it is now common practice to remove hair, all hair, from the pubic area following the industry belief that it makes one's genitalia appear larger, or that it dramatically enhances sensual effect. There are some generational as well as cultural divides here as well: pre-, post-, and up-to-date with the porn effect. Some older individuals have kept up with trends as influenced by the mass dissemination of free porn post 2008. Yet others, typically porn effect–naïve older individuals (re-entering the dating world from long-term monogamous relationships), can be shocked to find that pubic hair has gone the way of the dodo bird: they are facing dramatic mass changes in sexual attitude as well as sexual grooming. The younger have long been in the know and in the practice.

The effects do not end here. Now, fully exposed, increasing numbers of women, young and old, are having labial reconstruction surgeries and bleaching the skin surrounding their anus as there is now a more and a less desirable shape and coloration for these areas too. Men are also affected; older men, in particular, are having their testicles lifted to look younger than their testes would otherwise reveal. Apart from the age-old belief for men that bigger is better and now not-so-unusual surgeries for women involving sexualized areas that are partially visible through clothing (e.g., breast implants, lifts, and reconstructions), where do people get such ideas on such specifics as what such intimate areas of the body should look like? How do they spread so widely to normal dating or "non-professional" sexual culture? You got it, the Internet and the mass dissemination of porn. Today, everyone knows what someone should look like, not necessarily though personal experience or mass partners, but by the viewing of porn and essentially being told, and thereafter believing, and conforming, to an idealized form of sexual beauty dictated by an industry.

Porn Effects

We have known for quite a while that porn can have negative

effects on women's self-esteem (sexual, physical, and emotional). For example, women whose male partners view significant amounts of porn (and the women are aware of it) often develop confidence issues vis-à-vis performance and negative body image. This can result in altered sexual behavior including defensive decreased interest, requests for lights off, and even withdrawing from sexual activity entirely (indeed a most ironic catch-22 leading to compromised sex lives for both individuals). Some women develop an "if you can't beat 'em, join 'em" attitude, but the "positive" spin here tends to be short lived. Again, many women feel they are competing with, and being superseded by, an ideal: sharing a stage that should belong to them, and only them, within their partnership. But the playing field is evening. Increasing numbers of men now also suffer from confidence issues as a result of comparing themselves to the men on their screens. There is also a second effect too: arguably a purely Internet effect.

The aforementioned women's issues became magnified with the larger dissemination of men's magazines: what could be termed the *Playboy* or *Penthouse* effect in the 1970s. But they were inherent in unequal sexual/gender relationships throughout the ages wherein men openly or covertly went to strip clubs or brothels, or had mistresses. What I refer to as the "join 'em" effect is rather modern, and has exploded in the i-tech age. Pre-1960s (and some would argue much later), there was a social and stigmatic division between "good" women, AKA wives and mothers, and "bad" or wanton women, AKA prostitutes and mistresses or women willing to engage in premarital sex: not so much for men...

The sexual revolution for women now has a second, not so little, i-tech twist. In the next sections, I ask the reader to seriously ponder what the sexual liberation of women has morphed into in the digital age. Are we going forwards yet rather backwards?

Performance

Sexual performance and repertoire are grossly affected by the i-tech world. In the same vein as perception of beauty of genitalia, many people (predominantly female) are now offering more varied sex acts not because they necessarily want to, it feels better, or because they enjoy it more, but because this is perceived as what one should do, what others want and will react to positively. Equally disturbing from a clinician's perspective is the belief that mimicking extensive porn repertoire, acrobatics, vocalizations, and posturing (including feigning increased enjoyment of acts and arousal cycles) is the only way to stay in the game.

Many people feel they need to act like the Internet standard, as porn stars, or as the various amateur individuals posting their sexual exploits online for all to see. Many people now believe they need to compete with online activity to remain sexually desirable or sexually valid. This is concerning in adult culture but downright disturbing and destabilizing in adolescent culture.

The Converging of Desensitization and Disinhibition

Repeating my theme: we can't blame it all on the Internet and i-tech. The propagation of sexual imagery started long before and, in modern secular culture at least, has been steady increasing over the last few decades. It is not just the porn industry: the advertising, music, and entertainment industries are all equally guilty. We are bombarded with sex everywhere – in print ads, music videos, movies, television. Sex sells: thus near naked young people in highly suggestive, if not sexually overt, stances are everywhere, always in view, always selling something.

No one now bats an eye at the Victoria's Secret catalogue that caused such a scandal in the 1980s. The Angels and Guess girls and boys parade across our TV screens and pose seductively at our bus stops and in shop windows for all ages to see. The Internet has merely magnified and accelerated the process. We are now moving at lightning speed in terms of availability and exposure to all extremes of all forms of sexual content and process.

Sex may sell, but it is playing with the notion of desire in our brains in other ways too. There are a few more quite unexpected twists arising from the new dynamics of Internet sex. We are aware of the desensitizing effect: e.g., the more sex shown on TV, the less we react to it. But we forgot about desensitization's little cousin, arousal. Extensive unrelenting exposure to sexual content is affecting arousal templates.

Arousal Templates

An arousal template is simply a measurement of how much a person needs to see, hear, think of, touch, feel, smell in order to become aroused; due to i-tech, ours are getting higher. This is a principle known in addiction as raising the tolerance threshold. Tolerance is when, due to increased exposure, you need more and more for the same effect. You need more and more alcohol, cocaine, or heroin to get the same high. In the case of Internet sex exposure, you need to view or participate in more and more engaging or different content to become sexually aroused. It is not just a matter of more, however; it is a matter of what. Continuing with the addiction analogy, it is the requiring of alcohol, followed by marijuana, followed by cocaine, then heroin and crystal meth. You are not necessarily getting higher, but you need more or chemically stronger, or at the very least different, substances to get the same high or identical arousal. Back to sexual arousal thresholds: you need more even to be just plain interested.

The first twist to sex on the net is, at some point, real life stops competing; quite frankly it can't. The Internet is offering much more than typical, true, or real-life interpersonal human relationships, sexual and otherwise, can provide...or is it less? Let's start with more.

More

The Internet shows us more, much more than what occurs in the average person's life in an average week. With the obvious exception of actual touch from another, the Internet provides us instantly with more in every sense of the word, more positions, more orifices, more people (and other live creatures), more locations, more objects, more toys, more frequency, more size, more shapes, more material, more substance: just plain more visual everything. In cybersex it can also provide us with more communication wherein there is more intensity, more explicitness, more games, more availability, more tension, again more anything should you want it.

The resulting effect for many individuals is they now need this "more" to become sexually interested and, equally important, sexually responsive. With excessive online sexual engagement, arousal templates are being raised to the point that some individuals are no longer being sufficiently stimulated by real-life sexual experiences. Today, many individuals prefer the novelty, anonymity, and variety available online rather than potential for, or actual real-life prospects. They also prefer the instant availability, the instant "readiness."[180 181 182] Simply put, real-life sexual activity and the pursuit thereof is not as arousing or as intriguing as the content (fetish and otherwise) instantly available on the Internet. Obviously most people don't look "as good" as the people presented in porn but they also are not always as instantly interested, as ready, as aroused, as willing to "do anything" as found with a tap or the click of a button or of a mouse.

The resulting effect for many individuals is they now need this "more" to become sexually interested and, equally important, sexually responsive.

Less

Less will take a little more time to explain as it tramples directly on many of our written and unwritten moral codes: ones many of us want to believe we all wish to live by.

You may have noticed I have spoken of changes in perception of beauty and of process or performance crossing from the professional (or porn) world to the regular or offline world, but apart from the concept of "moreness" and effects on self-esteem, I have not as of yet spoken of emotions. Indeed, where have emotions gone in this new game of imagery and performance? Here yet another sexual profession enters the scene.

Internet porn and arguably many cybersex encounters are desensitizing in more ways than one. They strip away romance and intimacy, including expectation, desire, and curiosity of one person to truly explore another beyond the explicitness of the sexual process itself. In essence, i-sex is taking away the caress, both literally and figuratively.

For the masses, i-sex is stripping the sexual process of emotional process. There are no emotions other than those that play with arousal and arousal cycles. It gives you exactly what you want when you want it, and the majority of interactions or viewings have no strings attached – emotional or otherwise.

For the masses, i-sex is stripping the sexual process of emotional process.

There are no demands, no expectations, no compromises or sacrifices, no giving what you don't want to give, and certainly no receiving what you don't want to receive: nothing you usually get and receive from other people in intimate sexual relationships. And if there are, and you don't want them, you can simply click off.

We act differently and treat people differently online. This is in part because the medium itself thwarts our ability to read emotions by lowering our sensitivity to cues in facial expressions and voice prosody, but it is also because we just don't pay attention to them in our disinhibition. Some of it, however, is simply because we *can* not pay attention to the emotions of the other, that is. In sum, the medium directly promotes narcissism.

In many senses we don't view the other person(s) behind the keyboard, screen, or camera in the interaction as people at all, they are Internet people: people with whom, by context, the rules of engagement can be considerably different. Internet people do not have to know who you really are and all that implies regarding identity, personality, commitment, or duty. With Internet people you can click on and off, respond, delay response, or not respond at all: engaging and disengaging exactly when, and how, you want. If you don't like what you see or receive, you end it; you move on. Again this type of relationship is not new; in fact, it follows many of the rules of service, of shopping...of yet another sexual profession, of prostitution.

Momentarily setting principles of religion(s), morality, and such aside, one reason why prostitution remains popular is not because the majority of people would not be able to engage in sex otherwise, but rather that they would not be able to engage in precisely the emotional-sexual relationship that they want, or rather don't want (and when *they* want it).

Purchased sex, like Internet sex, although physically involving the touch of another body, does not have to have anything to do with romance, sharing, or intimacy; it is a completely narcissistic process. It's all about you, the customer, the consumer.

In the act, there are no true emotions, or conduct or performance expectations, including explicit judgment, demands for reciprocation, what to do, or not do, that are not pre-negotiated by circumstance or that you cannot immediately re-direct or remove yourself from if you are displeased. It is a performance solely for the benefit of the purchaser. There is also certainly no rejection. There is no "buzz off, slut," "as if, creep," "sorry, I'm not interested," "OK, but only after you buy me dinner and hold my hand," "not today," "no, not that way," "sorry honey, I have a headache," "the kids will hear us," "you just don't do it for me," or "we need to talk." You get precisely what you want, when you want it, or you move on to the next service provider.

Identically, online, if you get responses, reactions, or images you don't particularly want, or that don't arouse you the way you want, on you click to the next chat, person, or frame. In fact for many, this shifting, this searching, is part of the appeal, part of the intrigue.

Of note, for those of you who hold to the belief that the sex trade worker is actually in control and/or there is emotional sharing, both are still part of the business relationship. The way control is wielded and emotions shared (or mimicked) is part of the intended or desired dynamic in some sexual transactions. Manipulation, such as non-availability, not concluding sex acts, relationship mimicking, sharing of personal lives, pseudo sadism, etc., are explicitly part of some seller-buyer relationships: increasing desire and triggering specific desired emotional states of the purchaser.

That said, in prostitution (just as online), sometimes the emotional-sexual dynamic becomes enmeshed: affections, dependences, and other emotions can develop or evolve. But fundamentally it is exactly as the two (or more) players have agreed to within the situational context of the financial agreement. The individual purchasing always has final control by continuing or returning for more...or not.

In prostitution, control and emotional dynamics are often confounded with a business model. The sex trade operates like any other business. Take, for example, the food service industry or the retail industry. One restaurant serves filet mignon on white linen, the other burgers in waxed paper. One will serve any client regardless of comportment or attire, while others have no-shirt– no-service and even tie policies. For some transactions, by not giving purchasers what they want, the seller is giving them exactly what they want. A perfect example is that of snobby salespersons in exclusive shops: they want you to buy, their jobs depend on it, and their attitudes are sales tools that tend to sell more in the end. Equally, there are stores where a friendly attitude is central. In some businesses, clerks are even instructed to read a customer's first name off their credit card and accordingly "work the familiarity" or friendship angle at the till.

Even under idyllic circumstances (e.g., women and men who choose to use their bodies as commodities totally unaffiliated with sex trafficking, or with trying to escape personal histories of sexual and emotional abuse, coercion, extortion, mass poverty, drug addiction, and the like), the only control a sex trade worker has is in agreeing or not agreeing to work under certain conditions and with specific service attitudes – back to working in a burger house or a steak house or various forms of retail.

Now all that said, prostitution too is alive and well on the net, but that is an entire book on its own.

More...and Exactly What I Want

Now why all this explanation of the dynamics of prostitution? First, just like with sex for sale, despite multiple players, online sexual experiences are entirely individualistic: everyone is a John, a purchaser of sorts. And, as such, they follow John rules. Online sexual pursuits are mediated by a technology (rather than money) and, as outlined above, this results in entirely different rules of engagement and disengagement. A second parallel to prostitution is people do not suffer the same consequences of their actions or non-actions in this forum. As part of this, people can and do explore sexual pursuits in complete anonymity or relative fantasy, engaging in behaviors or experiences they never would otherwise in real life, again without the consequences one might find in said real life. As a participant in one of my studies wrote: "I also enjoy anonymity...it [the Internet] serves as an outlet for sexual fantasies that I would not do in person."

Women can and do play as men; otherwise straight men can play with men; much older women can seduce very young men – you can have as many and as varied experiences as you want sequentially or simultaneously. You can brag and boast, share select aspects of yourself, while simultaneously lying, hiding, or avoiding others. You can be crude, evil, and downright hurtful, or sensual and kind where words usually fail you – all this without the sometimes extreme emotional or social (and even legal) fallout when partners or strangers experiment with such things in body. Online, there is no social responsibility whatsoever. It is the ultimate fantasy and arguably pretty harmless, if it were not for the resulting altering of arousal cycles, and related alterations in socio-sexual emotive process in real life.

Shake Your Tail Feather: Everyone Gone Wild, or Gone Too Far?

Sexual Deviance

So where does this all leave us? What is normal? What is healthy? I frequently joke with friends and clients that the more educated I become, the more often I find myself answering "it depends," and this is definitely the case with sexuality and sexual practice. Definitions of healthy and normal sexuality, including sexual expression, curiosity, and exploration vary tremendously by culture, and, indeed the Internet is a culture. That said, for many, and certainly the younger generations, the culture has crossed over: boundaries of online and offline behavior again are becoming completely blurred, or should I say, are merging.

...boundaries of online and offline behavior again are becoming completely blurred, or should I say, are merging.

Through desensitization, the Internet is also normalizing what we used to refer to as sexual deviance. Sexual deviance, or the not normal, not healthy, or sometimes merely not usual, can be defined clinically, socially, or legally. It is also culturally (and historically) bound: what is deviant for one culture, or sexual couple, or group, may not be for another. Generally speaking, though, most cultures agree that it is sexual activity involving (unwanted) exposure, humiliation, pain, voyeurism, manipulation, extortion, minors or children, purchase and sale of bodies, and last but not least, deceit.

Infidelity

This last classification, deceit, is grossly affected by i-tech. The Internet is doing with infidelity (including cybersex, prostitution, and in-person affairs) what the advertising and music industries did for seduction. Through its propagation, infidelity is being normalized.

A Magnifying Glass or a Looking Glass?

That said, it is hard to get true numbers on activities that people tend to either boast about or want to cover up. Infidelity falls into this classification. Some cultures boast, and some hide, typically along a gender divide. Nonetheless, most infidelity is opportunity based, and the role of the Internet is in providing said opportunity, and lots of it.

Infidelity tends to be polarized: it is purely circumstantial or explicitly sought out. In the circumstantial, sparks have to fly at the office or the gym or wherever otherwise committed people spend enough time crossing for intrigue and interest to manifest. This can still happen with or without i-tech. What has changed, however, is the explicit seek and search method i-tech now facilitates. Prior to the Internet if an individual wanted an affair, he or she had to go out with explicit intent (e.g., to a bar or night club without their wedding ring) to attract another mate. The Internet has changed all this: opportunity, for everyone, is now literally at their fingertips.

The industry knows this and exploits this. Dating sites and infidelity sites now specifically cater to individuals wanting to cheat. Again availability is having a normalization effect. People in otherwise mutually agreed upon monogamous relationships who otherwise would not have gone out fishing for extramarital relationships are now doing so. The effects on pair bonding are catastrophic. Offline affairs and cyber affairs are increasingly common.

Regardless of the pre-post–Internet statistics on infidelity, and definitions thereof, the Internet is definitely directly responsible for the dissemination of acceptability. Case in point, agencies that would only be seen online are now starting to advertise mainstream. Explicit infidelity sites such as Ashley Madison are now advertising on television, and prostitution services (massage parlors) are now blatantly as opposed to covertly advertising in mainstream newspapers.

Very early on Shaffer (in 1996)[183] noted that increases in the prevalence of problematic Internet behavior were quite simply due to increases in accessibility. This indeed does appear to be the case in regards to online sexual practice. Due to increased accessibility, what we typically would refer to as "problematic behavior" has snowballed.

We are now a long, long way from a little harmless sexual exploration or fantasy. The disinhibition effect, resulting in disaffected arousal templates, disaffected pair bonding, precisely defined sexual performance and beauty expectations, and mounting preferences for Internet relationships (or non-relationships) and mere viewing with masturbatory practice are now increasingly superseding the desire for person-to-person sexual pursuits. Fewer people want people, intrigue, or discovery; they just want sex.

Brain Wiring and the Death of Intimacy

In my research on sexuality online[184] I tripped across a few other interesting factors. First, I confirmed that in contrast to popular belief, males and females engage in sexual pursuits relatively equally online. Females just happen to be less admissive or open about it. Second, similar to findings on television viewing, the viewing of sexual activity or erotica online actually reduces, not raises, the interest in and the performance of real-life sexual activity.[185] [186] [187] [188] Lastly, and this was the eye opener, in my study at least, this phenomenon was exclusive to males. In my study, 70% of males sexually engaging online reported "less interest in sex" and "almost no interest in sex." Not one of the females did. One of the explanations is that arousal templates are being affected. The other is that perhaps, for males, this is enough.

Why the difference?

With males and females, there is a difference in what we tend to do, or view, online. The activities females were mostly pursuing were relationship based, whereas males' activities were mostly pure objectification. This too makes for a frightening larger picture. Males tend to engage more through pornography, while females and gay males tend to engage though cybersex including role-playing games. Noted early in the cybersex phenomenon, females were seeking out sexual activities that involved romance, fantasy, and exhibitionism: in other words, interactive, or person-to-person activities. In contrast, males sought pornography, anonymity, and voyeurism.[189] [190]

As a popular saying in neurological studies goes, *neurons that fire together, wire together.* The findings of my research, and that of others, may indicate a cultural trend that sexuality for males is increasingly sought out and expressed online to the exclusion of real life. A discussion that may be worthy of further contemplation is the role of the de facto division of sexuality and intimacy provided by the medium, the Internet (as discussed in comparison earlier with purchased sex). Are men rewiring, becoming increasingly satisfied by objectified non-emotional sexual pursuits?

When pondering this question, I am particularly concerned about the preteen-teenage range of males, and the type of sexual beings they grow up to be. At a time when it is perfectly natural to be curious about sex and the opposite gender (for most), boys are increasingly exploring sex on the Internet. And, again, they are finding everything. More importantly, however, is what they are learning. Young males are learning what is available online, and this, not real-life girls, is defining what they expect and thereafter demand from future (or present) sexual partners, peers, or friends.

Again, real life can't honestly compete. First sexual experiences are terribly exciting but they are also typically awkward, as people explore and learn how to touch, talk, emote, give, take, and share their (hearts) and bodies. But boys have "learned everything" already, by Internet standards that is, and they expect, in fact need, girls to react the way the women do online to become interested or aroused. The double twist is girls know this and many now feel extreme pressure to compete or live up to the porn standard presented online.

Adolescents are now partaking in sexual games and "advanced" sexual repertoire that many, including myself, believe are not emotionally (or physically) healthy at this stage in life, including anal sex, group sex, and girls without lesbian tendencies or self-generated curiosity kissing or performing oral acts on each other not for their own pleasure, but to entertain boys who are watching. Again, i-tech is thwarting healthy socio-emotional sexual development. For adolescents and youth, the joy of sex may be gone, replaced by the performance of sex. Although I am not crazy about the religious framing of his work, one author, Struthers,[191] has some very powerful points in his book *Wired for Intimacy*. In this book, Struthers speaks about how when pornography is the model, sexual technique replaces sexual intimacy; we focus on the physiology, including the sensations of sexual acts and not the relationship(s) for which they are intended. His very valid thesis is that pornography corrupts intimacy. Looping back again to attachment, boys are not learning about what it means to be a man, and within this a sexual being, a lover, and potentially a partner, from their elders, including role modeling from fathers, uncles, or older brothers. They are learning from porn.

...boys are not learning about what it means to be a man, and within this a sexual being, a lover, and potentially a partner, from their elders.... They are learning from porn.

The frightening component for a therapist of my generation is it appears the early viewing of porn completely rewires many young males' sexual expression, including their sexual expectations and sexual desire. There has to be some sort of drive fueling sexual process and what we are seeing, at least in males, is the drive to pursue real-life sexual experience, unless dramatically explicit, is lessening and in many aspects absent. This is not only a matter of arousal templates, as discussed above, it is a matter of wiring: young males don't pursue females the way they once did. As such, and quite reactively I believe, females are now increasingly the sexual pursuers, offering more and more to be accepted or desired.

Naomi Wolf wrote a beautiful two-page article called "The Porn Myth"[192] synthesizing the phenomenon: how the mystery, the intrigue, and the exploration of sex was completely absent for the young. They just "do it" (sorry, Nike). She also wrote on the loss of feminine sexual power: how young women today have never experienced the pursuit and the power of their own sexuality and desirability therein. She also spoke to how the fears that accessibility of porn would turn men into raving sex maniacs were completely unfounded. In fact, i-tech has turned many into modern-day eunuchs, happy without the touch or heart of another, satisfying themselves with masturbatory practice, cybersex, and porn.

Bottom line, the novelty, variety, explicitness, and responsiveness online is higher, leading to young, and now many older males, becoming less and less interested or no longer aroused by real-life sexual experiences unless they are "competitive." They do explore real-life relationships, but then systematically return to the novelty, anonymity, and variety available online, which again fuels the cycle.

Back to Pathology

I have been speaking a lot of a void of emotion in sexual pursuits online. In one area, however, sexual pursuit is still all about emotion. Ironically, perhaps, it is in the realm of addiction. Sexual compulsion, or online sex addiction, paradoxically is rather fraught with emotion.

Addiction to pornography or cybersex has been found to be specifically related to depression and anxiety.[193] [194] [195] [196] Sexual process, like any process online, is fraught with anticipation and reward, and online sex addicts gorge themselves with these as a self-soothing mechanism.

For individuals who develop a compulsion, participating in online sexual pursuits is used as a mood regulator. Typically it is an avoidance technique, wherein individuals pursue their compulsion online to avoid real-life situations and to reduce anxiety. Like any drug, it calms them, temporarily at least.

For these individuals, building and being in control is extremely important in all the pseudo-relationships they construct online. Apart from the facility of availability, there is a reason why individuals seek out online relationships as opposed to in-person ones. They need this control, they need this validation.

Depending on where one is in the addiction cycle, there can also be what I refer to as compounding crossover. An individual may initially develop an online sexual compulsion due to the disinhibition factor but later lose the need for anonymity with the acceleration of the addiction. At a certain point, some individuals go offline, engaging in prostitution services, affairs, or encounters with individuals they meet through cybersex relationships. In sexual compulsion, the shedding of anonymity is part of the heightening process of addiction: part of the value to the increased physical stimulation and emotional soothing the individual is seeking.

Just as cyberbullying has been showcased in the media for its extreme potential for harm, so too sex addiction. As media, this time very accurately, portrays, the effects of both are often devastating. For professionals who work with many pathologies or processes affected by i-tech, it is very easy to remain over-objective, explaining or defining the process or the purposes they serve, just as I have above. In this we must not forget the human element, the human cost. When individuals (and not only those in partnerships) partake in this form of addictive process they kill the souls of many around them. As Linden wrote:

> If you are conscientious about using your drug of choice, it's possible to inflict pain mostly on yourself. By comparison, sex addicts by definition use other

> people and inevitably leave a wide swath of emotional destruction in their wake, severely testing the limits of compassion. (Linden, 2011)[197]

Sexual Mimicking

A lot of what I have been discussing falls under the framework of the blurring of sexual mimicking (from porn) with sexual experiencing with or without romance and intimacy. The age classes I have been discussing are adolescents through adults. But what about children, true children?

It seems with every passing decade, children are growing up faster. Innocence has been long lost with the aid of television and the music industry. Increasingly sexualized music videos for younger and younger audiences are more and more common. Case in point, ten or so years ago, at the height of Britney Spears and Christina Aguilera's careers (and very sexualized videos) their main following was tweens: nine- to twelve-year-old girls in fact.

How young women express themselves musically and sexually is irrelevant here: power to them. What is relevant is the effect on the intended or perhaps non-intended audience: how young girls mimic their idols, their way of dress, and their behavior. And by proxy how the rest of the world (e.g., boys in their peer group) start to expect girls to act too. What children see, children do, and the fallout I am seeing as a clinician is pretty scary. Bottom line, children between eight and thirteen are now far too sexualized.

Very Young Children and Sexual Mimicking

A few years back I would occasionally see a concerned parent who had discovered that his or her child was involved in early sexual exploration and was not quite sure what was appropriate. The games were usually the standard variations on "doctor" or "I'll show you mine if you show me yours." The therapy was very straightforward involving educating parents on the natural stages of healthy sexual development in children followed by the discussion of healthy or natural exploration within the boundaries of respect for self and others. Then I started seeing something different: a surge in what was being referred to as child sexual predators. Meet six-year-old Tylor.

Tylor's parents were in a panic and rightly so. It appeared that Tylor had been doing a little bit more than playing the game of look and touch with a little girl in the neighborhood. The description of the children's activities was full-on oral sex. When the little girl's parents found out about it, reaction was understandably extreme. So was the fallout. The result of the discovery was a public accusation of Tylor's family.

The accusation was on two levels: first that Tylor himself was being sexually abused (where else would he get such ideas other than from exposure or experience), and second, that Tylor was a budding sexual predator. What Tylor was, it turns out, was a child who had been exposed to pornography. Through play he was now mimicking the "pleasurable" behavior he had seen without any notions of right, wrong, appropriateness, or for that matter context.

Under such circumstances I ask you all for a moment to defer judgment on how and why Tylor got access to such material and instead look at the realities of accessibility in the digital age. Kids do not need to find their parents' or elder siblings' sites; they find their own or, more commonly, the sites find them. A child doing a school project on beavers will not find only information on swamp-dwelling, nest-building rodents. Pop-ups appear on children's computers too. Pornography is everywhere!

Tylor and his family barely survived this ordeal; they were humiliated, shunned, lost friends and family, chose to move from their neighborhood, and, yes, had a record of police investigation and social services involvement. What is this technology doing?

Sexting

Back to normal, I think...There is a new way we are staying sexually connected or is it sexually aroused: sexting. We fire little sexual messages and sexualized images at each other: some exploratory, some cute, some pretty explicit. This perhaps is just a tool and availability issue. Just like the keyboard changed availability and connectivity when compared to the pen, so too here.

Fifteen years ago, few of us would have left explicit sexual notes or pictures in our partner's lunch bags. Nor would we phone our spouses or boyfriends at the office to whisper sweet nothings or crude somethings into their ears with any regularity. The novelty would soon wear off, and continuing such practice would not have been considered typical, but rather perverse sexual behavior. But we now do. In fact, many people do, quite regularly, via text.

Are we now more sexualized? In the positive, are we now more in tune with our partners, sweetly reminding them they are desirable: keeping the sexual bond alive, strong? In the negative, is it part of the desperate need to perform to stay in the game? Is it an availability issue due to the ease of accessibility of the technology, or an expanding boundary issue, or is it just the new technological form of foreplay? Who knows, a point to ponder: the jury is still out.

The only area I would again ask parents to be cautious of is the practice with young teens. Teens who sext are sexualized, early. Meaning they act on the messages and pictures they send and receive (they also can share and post to devastating effect). Teens who don't partake in the process tend to wait a little longer, until they are a little older, to become physically engaged.

Community Solutions

What to do? Quite simply, take your sex life offline. For those of you with companions or spouses, get back to your bedrooms, kitchens, sofas, or wherever you can enjoy the company and body of your partner. Eat together, play together, let the sexual tension and desire build. Let the laundry pile

> Quite simply, take your sex life offline.

grow: intimacy, pair bonding, and harmony are more important than clean socks. Massage each other's feet, cook together, and when your nine-year-old wants to buy a thong because all the other little girls have them, say "hell no" and buy her the little girl panties she should be wearing until she is old enough to know why you don't want panty lines or the shape of your bum in your underwear is relevant to someone deserving. Only allow screen time in family rooms or put blocking and controlling devices on the children's computers; check those texts for sexts; and get on with real life!

For those of you single, get face to face and heart to heart. Turn off your i-tech occasionally when in company and alone; be with and explore the people around you. When in your own company, enjoy it, enjoy yourself: paint, sing, draw, read, play guitar, row, cycle, heck, play a game or two on i-tech (but limit the porn). Own your own time! You will be a much more interesting (and desirable) person for it. For men in particular, if you limit the porn, you will also perform better in person. Varying degrees of erectile dysfunction, including not being able to get or sustain a full erection and (unwanted) delayed orgasm in person-to-person contact is increasingly connected with masturbatory practice with porn.[198] And this is not the type of dysfunction Viagra and the like will help with.

Lastly, but very relevant in today's frantic world, when you feel stressed, depressed, bored, or lonely, resist reaching for porn, reach out to partners, and thereafter to family, friends, community, or clubs, less so to i-tech. If things feel desperate, seek professional help to bridge you. Going online for social and sexual purpose has directly been associated with exacerbation, not relief, of negative sentiment and disturbed affect (e.g., depression and anxiety). People need people, real people. If you don't feel you can handle people, and there are definitely times when one cannot and should not: go for a walk, hug a tree, punch a punching bag, get on your bike and fly. Get the energy out, but in a way that helps, not harms. This is not to say don't ever self-pleasure or masturbate, with i-tech or other; the Catholic priests lost that silly battle long ago. Just be aware of the brain wiring issue.

If you start to regularly prefer porn, web cams, or cybersex to regular offline people when people are available and desirous (with a little caressing) and/or your performance is not up to previous par, you have a pretty serious warning flag.

CHAPTER TWELVE

Community, Communication, Digital Mediation, and Friendship

Emotions and Language

First, something to think about.

When we look at the changes in our own behavior due to i-tech, the first thing to very seriously consider is that the whole concept of social media was thought up by an individual who many suspect has Asperger's: the characteristics of which are typically superior intelligence and interpersonal difficulties. The interpersonal difficulties many with Asperger's face are difficulty communicating; an inability to interpret social cues (including body language, vocalizations, and facial expressions) and perceive other's emotions; difficulty engaging in social routines; inability to see other people's perspectives; difficulty feeling or expressing empathy; difficulty forming friendships and intimate relationships; trouble interpreting social rules; problems regulating emotions typically manifesting in anger, anxiety, and depression; and a need for order.

Fine, genius in fact, for any individual, never mind one who may see the world atypically, to seed an entirely new digitally mediated social system that essentially mitigates against, and controls for, all of the above. A completely controlled social world that works quite well with punctuated smiley faces, "likes," kisses and frowns, all caps for emphasis, anger or yelling, winks for sarcasm. It is all perfectly clear, efficient: no emotive translation needed. Except that the primary social or communication system many of us (who in theory do not have atypical social perception) are now using was potentially launched from a brain that views socialization from an entirely different neurological platform.

I am not so much worried that we are occasionally functioning within the boundaries of a different emotive system. I am worried that we are all now increasingly operating from this different neuro-social platform, and suffering for it.

This is no longer theory. As directly evident in bullying and sexuality, the technology, and the space we are leaving it, is affecting the way we interrelate; we are expressing ourselves differently in the digital age. i-tech is altering not only our socialization style: it is altering our social process as well as our social processing. Every hour we spend on our computers reduces our interpersonal contact by one half hour and along with it our ability to interpret subtle nonverbal messages. It also makes us progressively socially awkward.[199] A study conducted on schoolchildren (in the sixth grade) found that children who were systematically on digital screens (as well as watching television) were compromised in reading human emotions. When compared to children who went on an i-tech and TV hiatus for only five days, children who continued to engage with digital devices, as per normal, had decreased abilities to understand the emotions of others as well as decreased sensitivity to emotive cues.[200] The conclusion drawn by this study and many others is that replacing person-to-person social interaction with i-tech and screen-mediated interaction reduces our social skills as well as our general well-being (happiness). I simply argue it reduces our observation skills, which affects all the above.

...children who were systematically on digital screens were compromised in reading human emotions.

You don't have to be a scientist or a psychologist to realize the concerning implications of a generation or two with reduced abilities to read human emotions. Reducing social skills, reducing the ability to understand emotions, reducing sensitivity to emotional cues, reducing inhibition, desensitizing us: is i-tech manufacturing autistic and Asperger-like symptoms in the masses? If we can't read each other, how can we care, empathize, come to each other's aid, love each other? Is i-tech desocializing us or just plain making us less human?

A New Language

As will be discussed in the next chapter, the medium now supports a whole new culture, but here I will speak to a whole new language: texting, or should I say txt. In fact, how to script was a big decision I had to make when writing this book. Would it be important for my readers, especially the younger ones, to script in the language of the times I am discussing? In the end, I chose the traditional; context indeed is critical. Text it is; this is a book after all. That said, I do argue, we, the older, should notice and partake in using the new scripting style when, and where, appropriate: for example, when scripting on our phones.

Change (and resistance) is nothing new in the evolution of written language. Just as our foremothers and forefathers resisted and then adapted to simplified grammar, contractions, and acronyms, so too should we to text or txt talk. As Tom Chatfield explores in his new book, *Netymology*,[201] there is a wealth of information in this new on-screen language. Older and formal educators do themselves a cultural disservice by resisting; indeed we will be left behind.

As Chatfield rightly points out, texting is a language for the eyes not the ears. It is not a degeneration of language; it's just different, substantially different. Texting involves frequent subtle changes in letters or format, that only the eyes (or perhaps braille) can see. For example an "s" shifting to a "z," choosing a small as opposed to a capital letter, variation in standard acronyms, and the creation of new ones provide not so subtle changes in messages or to a strength of phrase. Understanding these subtleties further speaks to youth culture and inclusion or non-inclusion in specific groups. In many ways it is the not-so-secret language of the young. And if the older do not partake, so it will exclusively evolve.

Functional-Emotive Crossover: Points to Ponder

So text talk is a different language, and, as with all languages, different expressions have different function. Or is it different functions have different expression, different emotion? Back to the autistic connection (e.g., an inability to express or interpret emotion) or the digital native connection (e.g., a new shallowness of phrase or thought we the older now see in the young): one question I do have is regarding the explicit function of symbols such as ☺ or ☹ or progressive emotive letter phrases such as lol, LOL, ROFL or ROFLMAO. Does this text talk speak to the brilliance of a new code in its conciseness or rather a need for translation of a language within a language? Is this brilliant layered complexity, of a sort we have never seen before, or a language that due to its shallowness cannot speak for itself without emotional or emphatic stage direction?

Points to Ponder in the Evolution of Digital Language

There are many and multiple facets or components to i-tech language and communication, including the sub-conversation, the parallel conversation, and, as explained above, layered or embedded meaning wherein format itself has connotation.

Sub-conversations and language layering are not at all new in the evolution of language. They are in fact rather common in multilingual environments. I was blessed myself to be able to experience this long before the advent of i-devices. When living in Europe as a young woman, I very much enjoyed the layering of language that naturally occurred when smaller communities or groups of friends spoke several languages. Depth and twists on meaning were delivered by, or accentuated by, language choice. A specific word in English would mean something slightly different in French, and entirely different in Italian. The same word repeated in two languages would underline meaning. One would both consciously and unconsciously choose the language of delivery accordingly. I terribly missed this when moving back to North America. One language was limiting.

Enter text talk. i-tech has brought this not so new feature to all of us, to the masses. As outlined above, the way one chooses to alter a word or phrase through pseudo or new "spellings," as well as emphatic, emotive, and otherwise meaning conveying formatting, indeed can create subtle but very distinct differences. With texting one can very efficiently selectively make meaning deeper, more precise, and yes exclusive. Which brings me to a second feature, the sub-conversation. Again, prior to i-tech, this was a feature exclusive to multilingual individuals. Polyglots, fully knowing what languages people do or do not speak, switch languages accordingly. This can be done to not interrupt conversation flow, for example switching languages at dinner party to ask for the bread basket, make a relevant but off-topic comment for select ears only, or to redirect children without drawing the specific attention of others at the table.

Some language switching can also be intentionally exclusive: one can animate a conversation, or express a view one does not want certain others to hear or understand. When working with families, at the clinic, I see this happen all the time. Clients will switch to a mother tongue, say Cantonese or Punjabi, which indeed

I do not understand, when they wish to express something amongst one another they do not want me to understand.

This switching is now regular practice with i-tech and digital natives. But as opposed to being linguistically mediated, conversation(s) and sub-conversation(s) are technologically mediated. There is common conversation usually verbal, as well as sub-conversation usually digital. If not malicious, nothing wrong with it: it is an interesting linguistic evolution, one everyone (not just polyglots) can now access. If fact, many digital immigrants strongly hold to the opinion that it can make an evening or experience more fulfilling, broader. Many older digital immigrants, however, miss the positive potential of this unique feature, complaining of rudeness, or that focus is negatively divided. I believe it simply boils down to what each of us is used to, and therefore what we can understand, without feeling threatened.

Regardless of language (digital or otherwise), unilingual individuals can feel threatened, multilingual ones less. Otherwise multilingual individuals in polyglot environments who do not speak a language spoken do not tend to get offended; if a point is important, they trust it will be translated, and, in my experience, it usually is. Much the same with on- and offline conversations: individuals will bring those present into what is being communicated on i-devices if they deem it important.

Back to spoken language only: individuals who demand that all conversations should be "inclusive" in the language they understand tend to be naïve as to the larger perception that they are being imperialistic in nature. For example, if I told my clients to speak in English only in my office, it speaks more to my need for control than my need to understand. There are of course exceptions, where language is used intentionally as a barrier, or intentionally as an exclusion or manipulation feature: same too with i-tech devices. Many individuals take advantage of this, intentionally ignoring or choosing to follow their i-devices as opposed to being present with others.

Enter the parallel conversation. Parallel usage is quite different from the sub-conversation. Here attention is indeed divided. Here too my digital immigrant status is evident. I, and those of my generation, often do not like competing with i-tech: we find it destabilizing, even insulting, to be in a verbal conversation as the person we are communicating with is seemingly only half present. A key difference, I believe, between the activity, and hence the emotional reaction, is the sub-conversation is intermittent adjunct, whereas the parallel conversation is constant, and hence competitive.

Our reactions may all come down to a game of numbers and frequency. In otherwise one-on-one interaction, individuals will feel superseded by i-tech if used too often or interrupting the flow of presence. At a table of twelve, or at a party, does it really matter; does the behavior have such an impact?

At dinner, children text and snap chat "under the table" much as they used to play games such as footsie, or make secret faces at each other twenty-five years ago. It was a sub-activity to eating and being with their elders. When adults had had enough, or the sub-activity became too dominant, they would reprimand children or ask them to stop. Other children just play i-games, stream, or surf, otherwise totally absent apart from occupying the same physical space as their siblings or parents.

A young woman at a restaurant today does not have to "politely" take her girlfriend to the bathroom or "rudely" whisper and giggle in her ear to tell her that she finds a fellow joining them intriguing. She texts across the table. She can also do the same for negative purpose, e.g., to criticize another young woman's dress or say she thinks she is a skank. She can also chat with her sister in Toronto while eating dinner with a friend in Vancouver. Again, it is not the technology that makes a situation positive or negative: it is how each of us chooses to wield it.

In essence there are multiple arguments, all relevant, all holding truth: all of which can be twisted or abused. Individuals can indeed be very rude, ignoring individuals present for conversations or searches via i-tech, leaving others annoyed, feeling there was or is, no purpose to gathering. Equally, individuals can be invasive in their demands for exclusive attention. It really truly boils down to attitude and context. I believe we are currently actively negotiating these boundaries. Integration versus interference, here perhaps, is a little harder to differentiate.

All this said, as will be discussed in the following section, there is something disquieting about disrupted energy flow: being present yet not. And we are all feeling it. Perhaps there is some formula to balance we have yet to discover.

A Game of Touch and Numbers

Feeling a Little Lonely and a Lot Agitated

Other books speak to feelings of social isolation in relationships due to the prevalence of online relationships and the dominant form of communication not being interpersonal at all.[202] Being on Facebook is quite simply not "being there," face to face, heart to heart. There are many studies that speak to the increased incidence of depression due to over-socialization online. Bottom line, the illusion of friendship via social networks and social sites, for many, leaves us feeling emptier, not fuller. It is not a fair trade or true substitution for live interpersonal interaction.

Even when we are together, sitting next to each other, many of us still feel alone, as attention is consistently on i-tech rather than on each other, and many of us are guilty. I once was working with an adolescent who called out her mother, who was lamenting about her excessive computer use and lack of interaction with family. As the parent was admonishing and lecturing her daughter, her daughter, with true and direct annoyance, snipped back, "What do you expect me to do? You are always on your computer." Again the feeling we often get with i-tech, even when in close physical proximity to others, is the person is "there but not there" and, more often than not, also not aware.

Other factors, however, affect how we think and act in our

otherwise interpersonal relationships. i-tech is changing more than our face-to-face patterns: it is changing our "belonging requirements."

Many individuals feel distressed and even panicked when they forget their phones at home, unable to focus on anything other than what they may be missing that would be communicated by the device. Others check their phones routinely, cannot even go to the bathroom without them. Dr. Rosen, in his book *iDisorder,*[203] collected some interesting statistics on this: 49% and 56% of the last two generations check their text messages "all the time." My generation (Gen X) and the one before (the Baby Boomers) check 34% and 17% respectively. And, at the time of this research this was only text, not social media, not news feeds, alarms, nor work email and all the other information streams now accessed by cell phones. This is a peculiar dependence on micro contact. Further, for many, the distress, including feelings of agitation, and anxiety they experience without this constant contact, culminates in panic attacks. The fear of missing out (now acronymed to FOMO) rules their conduct. And this "new disorder" too is on the rise.

Part of this is due to speed of information: the lack of "staying with something." Events and issues flash by and are not repeated or expounded upon; indeed they can be missed when one is not watching or present. The larger question I am asking us to truly examine as a culture, however, is are we really so connected due to our technology, or is it exactly the opposite: are we actually so disconnected that we need a device to ensure we are not alone, not left out?

...are we really so connected due to our technology, or is it exactly the opposite: are we actually so disconnected that we need a device to ensure we are not alone, not left out?

Distal and Proximal Relationships

This brings up other questions such as what is a friend and how many can we really have? There are some interesting studies on animal social groups: how they maintain friendships and how they keep the status of them. In other primates, for example, this is done through grooming, through touch. Grooming, for humans and other primates alike, however, is logistically limited, as beyond family itself, we only have so much time to groom each other; therefore we can only have so many friends.[204]

It is believed that humans were able to expand to larger social groups though variation in communication and ritual, primarily through laughter and through dance, permitting the bonding of larger groups. Still, it appears no true friendship circle can have any depth after growing past fifty. Quite simply, we may feel good together (laughing or dancing or talking) but we cannot get to, or keep any depth, of communication or emotion. As humans we cannot follow or "groom" a group that exceeds fifty. We are not fulfilled when our care or attention, or that of others, becomes too broad.

I question whether we are now experimenting with another social expansion. Are we in an unconscious social experiment that, for many of us, may be failing due to magnitude and, quite simply, lack of touch? It comes back to functional versus dysfunctional usage relating to functional and dysfunctional relationships. How and when, and to exclusion of what and whom, do we use or do not use technology (as discussed in Chapter Two)? What are we losing when we follow our 800 Facebook friends for five hours as opposed to having six friends over for a dinner party for the same period of time? What are we losing when we watch porn and masturbate to a multitude of images as opposed to make love, or, hell, have raw sex, with a person we care for? Gaming and social media are now undeniably tools of social bonding, but is the difference between functional bonding versus dysfunctional usage leading to emotional deregulation simply a question of group size and group proximity?

We know the two boys who play a computer game side by side are actually bonding whereas the ones playing across the country in MMOs are seeking the bonding, getting the illusion, but may not actually getting it, hence deregulating, feeling worse for it.

Similarly, adolescents on a subway train can be bonding with i-tech and feeling good while the one being communicated to distally can experience FOMO: not feeling the comfort of the reaching out, but rather the discomfort of lack of physical presence, triggering the "missing the party" effect, the anxiety, the loneliness, and the endless loop of texting.

This is not exclusive to digital media. Promoted by media itself, many of us are developing atypical relationships, or rather atypical perception of them. Just as we are increasingly relating and bonding to individuals we know only through i-tech, we are increasingly relating and bonding to individuals we know only through programming. For example, we are starting to feel we are friends with television and radio hosts, especially when presented in a group format. Delusional, well, not quite: we are being prompted to react this way. More social psychology...

The Role of Self-Revelation

When talking about social or political issues, individuals self-reveal, meaning they also talk about their children, their friends, boyfriends, or spouses, in intimate details, we emotively react. This response is quite natural, what humans are again designed to do. The catch is, once again, in such format, we don't "inter-react." It is an illusion. We are voyeurs not participants, and voyeurs typically either get pumped by secret knowledge, or they long to be a part of it, again feeling empty, wanting more. In pathology this can even turn into stalking.

i-tech again has a solution to this: Twitter. Twitter, email, Facebook postings, and the like streaming on shows give us just enough to feel belonging through participation. But again, in the big emotive picture, it leaves us empty.

Why media is doing this is obvious: loyal followings bring up ratings and have the side benefit of also loyally following politics and loyally buying products, but why are we buying in, literally and figuratively? Apart from marketing genius, I believe it once again is a need for belonging that we are no longer feeling in our primary relationships: a replacing of true intimacy with artificial intimacy.[205] Otherwise, in mediums supposedly designed to bring us together, why do we end up feeling so agitated or so alone?

Again, the phenomenon is not "generated" by i-tech, but rather exploited by it: we, the general public, always had this attraction to celebrity or public personas, be it rulers of old such as kings and queens, the superbly wealthy, movie stars, evening talk show hosts, etc. We admired them for their power, their talent, their position in life, which appeared superior to ours. The difference between then and now, however, was that we idolized them distally, we knew they were not of "our group"; we might mimic them but we were never so pretentious as to pretend we were, or would ever be, one of them. We were not "familiar" with them.

CHAPTER THIRTEEN

i-Addiction: A New World

So what is belonging? What is community? What are friends? How do we now define each in the digital age? Online social networks definitely have a place – and a positive one. Some friendships would not exist if it were not for the digital age. They would not bloom or be maintained; others would have long faded. For my generation and older, finding and reconnecting with long lost friends from childhood and youth was the greatest of pleasures and would not have been possible if not for Hotmail and Facebook. For all generations, keeping contact with people met on travels is equally lovely. Long distance relationships are also increasingly common, and significantly more successful than in the past due almost entirely to the ability to stay connected, bonded, through i-tech. There is no debate here; there are unequivocally benefits for the propagation and maintenance of distal relationships and networks of people expanded over physical space. But, for some, it has crossed over. The realm of i-tech is not just a new space that allows for the extension of boundaries of communication and the maintenance of distal relationships; it is a new space, or rather a new world, one in which they live and rather exclusively I might add.

Socialization Online: Another Dimension, Another World

The Internet has been described in popular literature as another country: a country with its own culture, its own communities, and even its own currency (e.g., Bitcoin). Some communities (e.g., in MMORPG games) even self-regulate, developing their own policing systems. For example, forums are set up wherein individual players can be banned from play for excessive aggressive or insulting language. There are also now online courts (e.g., eQuibbly.com in Canada and Swiftcourt out of Sweden),[206] with legal binding judgments. Individuals dissatisfied, deceived, or who otherwise feel jilted with products purchased online can now also litigate, and otherwise seek justice online with the services of online lawyers.

For the majority of Internet users, joining Internet communities through regular chat rooms, games, and the like is just good fun or more practical for work. The Web is merely an additional form of communication, entertainment, a research forum, etc.; we otherwise continue with positive social, familial, and work relationships. Second life really is a second place where people play, not a second place they "live." World of Warcraft is an interactive fantasy world, never confused with reality. For others, however, the Internet does confound, becoming an escape or obsession. The games take on new dimensions that fulfill empty emotional places or start to supersede offline relationships. Some individuals, regardless of gaming practice, also live their lives almost exclusively online. So who are these people so enmeshed? If the Internet is indeed another country, another world: who are its citizens?

Profiles

Initially, excessive individual Internet use and exclusive Internet communities were dominant in adolescent and university culture.[207] [208] Excessive usage was also inversely related to age and education.

The younger and more educated you were, the higher the likelihood that you had an obsessive relationship with the Internet. By 2011 it was estimated that from 6 to 14% of all adults had a significant Internet problem. Depending on your age and where you lived, this number could be as high as 38%. In South Korea and China, for example, Internet addiction in youth had reached epidemic proportions and was labeled a serious public health issue by 2008.[209 210]

A follow-through misconception from these early times was that excessive and enmeshed usage was a male issue. Not true: such usage is now equally predominant in males and females. A few interesting factoids, however, are that there are fewer females in treatment centers and they are generally a little more covert about their behavior. In games and such, many women also play cross gender. Because a lot of excessive female usage also tends to be in the realm of social networking and social gaming, it is also publicly perceived as less problematic. The effect on work, family, spouses, etc., however, is equally damaging; excessive focus on texting and social media over work, duty, family, or the individuals present, over time, has a cumulative toll.

Bottom line, the stereotype of the nerdy or introverted i-addict being a young man has not been accurate for a long while. There are now many niche profiles. As mentioned in Chapter One, retirees of both genders and newly separated or divorced mature females are currently one of the highest at-risk groups. Individuals in life transition or those who are feeling disenfranchised (e.g., adolescence), or who actually belong to a disenfranchised community (e.g., LGBT in small communities) are also at significantly higher risk. Why? Because for select individuals, the online world is a place where an otherwise compromised feeling of belonging can be found. Individuals can develop social networks that would otherwise not be available, and, at the click of a button.[211]

Now in 2014–15 there is yet another profile, youth who are failing to launch. These are older adolescents and young adults who almost literally get trapped online in their parents' basements.

They are typically under- or unemployed, playing with notions of going to school or career choices, but otherwise overwhelmed with choice or apathy (procrastination) leading to not taking the necessary steps to have their future manifest. They are supported by family, disability checks, or social services. They are trapped in enabling dynamics and frequently develop severe depression or anxiety. They use i-tech to entertain and distract and do not progress to the next natural or healthy stages in life. This is what Cassandra, presented in Chapter Six, was at risk of becoming.

So how do we know how much is excessive usage? Moving beyond technological interference, and sub-clinical pathologies, what is i-addiction and when do we know we have a problem? But first what is addiction?

Addiction – Classic Definitions

Addiction is a broad-based term. It is generally defined as a dependency on a specific chemical or narcotic substance such as alcohol or cocaine or to a behavior such as gambling, sexual activity, or eating.[212] An official diagnosis of addiction requires a compulsive pathological component that is destructive to self, work, school, or relationships.

Scientific Corner: The DSM-IV (a manual used by many psychologists and psychiatrists) defines addiction as "a cluster of cognitive, behavioral and physiological symptoms indicating that the individual continues use of the substance despite significant substance related problems" (DSMV-IV-TR. APA, 2000, p. 192)[213]. In this manual, behavioral disorders such as compulsive gambling are defined as "persistent and maladaptive behavior disrupting personal, family or vocational pursuits" (DSMV-IV-TR. APA, 2000, p. 671). Similarly binge eating addiction is defined as "recurrent episodes associated with subjective and behavioral indicators of impaired control over, and significant distress about the action" (DSMV-IV-TR. APA, 2000, p. 785). The American

Society of Addiction Medicine defines addiction as "a primary, chronic disease of brain reward, motivation, memory and related circuitry" (ASAM, 2011, para. 3).[214] Dysfunction in brain circuitry results in the biological, psychological, spiritual, and social traits associated with the maladaptive use and pursuit of substances or behaviors (ASAM, 2011). To sum this up, the simplest definition of addiction is: a malfunction of reward circuitry in the brain.

i-addiction definitely fits. It is a behavioral addiction affecting our relationships, our school or work, our brain circuitry regarding reward, motivation, and learning. It also affects our mood state and is highly linked with agitation. We choose it over partners and work, we binge compulsively on movies and shows, it leaves us with mood disorders like depression, and regulation issues such as anger when asked to disengage, and it creates generalized anxiety and insomnia.

As Dr. Orzack[215] defined it very early on (in 1999), i-addiction is a problem of impulse control. Despite clear negative consequences, we cannot disengage from the activity. Different from all but eating disorders, however, it has a little catch. Just as with food, abstinence from the technology is not a plausible alternative. Given the Internet's dominant role in our culture, as with food addictions, individuals must learn to regulate as opposed to eliminate behaviors. As such, it is significantly harder to manage. This form of addiction also leaves us with many questions, such as is it really the Internet itself? Is it the process or is it the pornography, the gambling, or the shopping available online that is the true addiction? How do we classify it: by content choice, by co-morbid trait, by degree?

Theories and Classifications of Internet Addiction

Until recently, it was fairly common to classify i-addiction by activity.

Block for example classified IA by three subtypes: communication (e-mail and texting), sexual preoccupation (pornography and sexual communication), and gaming (and sought inclusion of these classifications for the DSM-V).[216] From my perspective, there is potential for blurring across and within categories that may warrant a different classification structure. From my clinical perspective, classifying does not explain the role of process or why individuals find specific Internet activities appealing or addictive. Defining addiction by activity may limit our understanding of the phenomenon.

Scientific Corner: Of note, IA was typically categorized as a compulsive-impulsive spectrum disorder and was under consideration by the American Psychological Association for inclusion in the current DSM, the DSM-V (see Block, referenced above; Young, Yue, & Ying, 2011[217]). Gaming was the only classification to gain inclusion on its own.

What is unique to i-addiction is it often expands beyond a specific classification or choice of activity: the method, or medium of access itself, is central to the addiction.[218] At its core, Internet addiction involves both a behavior and the technology that facilitates the behavior. In this sense the Internet itself can be viewed as the environment or the condition that triggers and thereafter sustains the addictive behavior. And, as outlined earlier, we all feel the pull.

In i-addiction, however, the way an individual uses the medium (e.g., avoidance, disinhibition), as opposed to the content sought via the medium (e.g., social communication, pornography), also speaks to the nature or "purpose" of the addiction. It may be the medium as opposed to the content of the medium that is the true addiction.

It may be the medium as opposed to the content of the medium that is the true addiction.

Now, all that said, ask the spouse of one who is watching excessive porn and a hundred-to-one, there will be problems with content too, and obviously pedophiliac viewing (child porn) and other significant deviances are in classifications to themselves. But to larger society, as well as to the individuals themselves, in fact, no: what we are doing online is not as relevant as one might think. As already discussed with sexual addiction, there are associations with specific interests and specific pathology (which further may have treatment implications), but for the larger classification of i-addiction, however, "what" you are doing online is secondary to "why" you are online.

In 2012, I conducted an extensive exploration of scholars' writings on the subject. Streaming though the dominant perspectives on i-addiction, and their associated user or abuser profiles, I saw that three distinct themes and user types emerged. I classified them as Generalized Internet Addiction (GIA), Fantasy Internet Addiction (FIA), and Technological Internet Addiction (or TIA). And they really speak to the "why" not the "what" of excessive online usage.[219]

Generalized Internet Addiction

The first perspective I put together is that there is no IA per se. Excess Internet use is not an addiction in itself but rather, the Internet is the space where an individual can engage in the addictive behavior. The addiction is gambling, gaming, sex, shopping, and so forth. The Internet is merely the medium.[220] For example, a compulsive gambler can and will go to a casino, a private game, or the Internet. Equally, with compulsive shopping, the individual will go out and shop in actual stores or shop from home or work in online stores. For sexual compulsion, the individual will have virtual cybersex or engage in physical sexual contact with other individuals. For this first category, the fact that an individual chooses the Internet as the preferred tool of engagement is absolutely irrelevant.

Fantasy Internet Addiction

The second voice in the literature considers that the technology is intrinsically intertwined with the addiction. The individual would otherwise not engage in the activity if it were not accessible by this specific medium. This form of IA is directly related to anonymity, the shedding of self or the development of new or different self-identity. It falls under the category of fantasy wherein individuals typically develop another persona and role-play as this persona, for example, role-playing games such as Second Life or chat rooms and websites that promote virtual affairs and sexual experiences under pseudonyms. A key component in this form of addiction is the disinhibition offered by said anonymity.[221] The online disinhibition effect allows for individuals to shed their real persona and act differently. As presented in the section on sexuality and cyberbullying, the Internet offers different rules of engagement wherein consequences can be avoided and individuals can explore aspects of behavior or personality they would never otherwise do in real life.[222] In this second category, the individual gambler or sexual addict would not venture out in the non-virtual world. The gambler would not go to the casino and the sexual addict would not seek real-life sexual interaction, preferring instead the fantasy or the anonymous component offered by the medium, the Internet.[223] This second form of IA would be classified as a contextualized addiction as individuals limit themselves to experiences or behaviors that would not be available if not for an i-tech device.

Technological Internet Addiction

The third category can be classified as a pure technological addiction. For this third category, the structural component of the medium and the software combined are central in providing the properties that support addiction. Greenfield[224] identified these as searches or activities that function on a variable reinforcement schedule. They are identical to the rewards provided in traditional gambling addiction as they are unpredictable in both frequency and saliency.[225] When content and process are combined with a variable ratio reinforcement schedule, as well as 24-hour access and potential for increasingly stimulating content, it can be viewed as the perfect context for the development of an addiction. Gaming, gambling, stock watching and trading, e-mailing and texting, auction shopping, as well as pornography are all addictions that can be driven by both content and process as supplied by the medium, the Internet. This last classification appears to be the classification of most threat. Technological addiction is all about process, and more and more of us are succumbing to it.

To further understand the phenomenon, I conducted a study wherein I asked many questions on patterns and choices of activities of individuals who self-identified with being i-addicts. As expected, I found rather uniformly that individuals' activities and activity choice were not exclusive nor were they static. People were engaging in multiple activities and activity choices would change over time. For example, one woman indicated on the questionnaire that in the past she engaged extensively in fantasy gaming, but not so much now. Her choice of activities had broadened. For one young man, pornography was an activity he partook in often but definitely not exclusively. He enjoyed many other online activities. The findings from my study suggested that the process provided by the medium was equally if not more important than the chosen activity in the development of the addiction. This supports the very early position of Greenfield that the addiction expands beyond a specific classification or choice of activity. Greenfield as well as Shaffer stated early on in the phenomenon that the method or medium itself was central to the addiction.

Searching: Going Down the Rabbit Hole

A specific category of Internet usage that is not often discussed in relation to addiction is searching. The classification of searching may have initially received little attention, as for many individuals searching was one of the primary and non-problematic forms of Internet usage. It also does not carry any stigma as with sexual preoccupation and to a certain extent gaming. That said, searching is a major category of usage that is easily overtly or covertly masked or clouded by legitimate work-related and study-related activities. This clouding perhaps renders it even more insidious. When conversing with the participants in my study, it became very clear that although they were engaging in multiple classifications of usage, the category of searching was the dominant problem. One hundred percent of my participants reported using the Internet compulsively for searching. While I was chatting with participants about their experience of the process, an analogy that came to mind was that the searching process was rather akin to going down the rabbit hole in the tale *Alice in Wonderland*. Individuals jump in having no idea where they are going beyond into a hole in the ground following the proverbial white rabbit (the initial topic selected). They then find themselves immersed in a virtual Alice in Wonderland scenario completely incapable of getting out while simultaneously intrigued by unknown adventure (images and information) including the occasional re-appearance and opportunity to chase said white rabbit (the initial purpose of the search). Themes of "getting caught," "escaping," and "following information trails" were evident in both participants' written comments as well as what they shared in debriefing thereafter. This finding again speaks to how process may be equally if not more important in allure than content for the individual with IA.

Practical Ways to Assess When We Have a Problem (and Limitations)

When the issue of excessive and detrimental usage first started coming on the clinical radar, we did not have adequate tools to assess or prove to ourselves and others that indeed, for some, excessive usage was a problem. We all had our views; mine are presented in Chapter Two. Dr. Young, however, was the first to design a test to help concretely determine when Internet usage turns from neutral or inclusive to negative. Dr. Young's test (the IAT or Internet Addiction Test)[226] [227] specifically measures the extent of use as well as the level of interference in an individual's personal, professional, or scholastic life. The test specifically measures dependency. Dependency, in this context, is the effect of usage of i-media on an individual's functionality and their mental and physical health.[228]

Scientific Corner: Called the Internet Addiction Test or IAT, Dr. Young's test is the first (validated psychometric instrument) that measures addictive behavior as specifically related to computer utilization. The test measures non-academic and non-professional computer use and has been found by other scholars to be a reliable measure of pathological Internet consumption (see Ferraro, Caci, D'Amico, & Di Blasi, 2007,[229] Kazaal et al., 2008;[230] Widyanto and McMurren, 2004[231]).

The test measures four dimensions and six factors believed to be integral to the identification of Internet Addiction (or Digital Process Addiction). The four dimensions are interference with family relationships, salience and withdrawal, overindulgence in online relationships, and lastly tolerance and neglecting daily routines. The six factors are salience, excessive use, anticipation, lack of control, neglecting work, and neglecting social life.

The test can be found and taken online, and will place you in one of 4/5 categories from normal/healthy usage to problematic and addictive behavior. For those of us still engaged with work, school and social lives, the test is a very good indicator of levels of disengagement from community life.

So Far Gone That Assessment Fails

We may, however, have moved beyond this.

While seeking out participants for my i-addiction study, I used the IAT as a means of selection. This was the test with the track record. While recruiting, however, I noticed many of the candidates, who were clearly identifying with having a severe i-addiction, were systematically not scoring high enough on the test to be considered for inclusion. They were not "severe enough." As the IAT had proven its validity in numerous studies, and denial, not admittance, is the standard pattern in most addictions, I started to question if something was amiss.

The lovely thing about individuals with an i-addiction is they are rather communicative online. In email banter, people offered a lot of helpful information on their Internet patterns and the effect on their lives, further raising my suspicion that something was clearly wrong. I had an enigma. Now intrigue is something every researcher enjoys, except when it is completely mucking up their research plan.

Closely examining the situation, the only thing I found obvious was that these potential participants were single. I could let it go, but I did not want my study to be biased toward people in relationships. And then bingo! A potential participant gave me the answer in black and white. These individuals were scoring low because the test involved other people's opinions. And there were no other (offline) people in their lives to give opinions!

> A lot of questions "did not apply" because they involved someone else's opinion on how I spend my time and I do not have that kind of relationship with anyone, where they would judge/ask how I spend my time.

What I had haphazardly discovered though this "rejection" process is there are now manners of usage, or lifestyles in fact, that are so enmeshed with digital media that offline life is secondary, quite secondary, so much so that assessing the effect of i-tech on relationships is now a moot point. Questions regarding how Internet usage affected relationships legitimately did not apply. The interesting factor, however, was that this was not because Internet usage did not interfere with said existing offline relationships, rather that these relationships did not exist! And this was quite an eye opener.

A New Profile

For individuals who do not have, or for whatever reason never had or have lost, invested offline personal relationships (e.g., living alone, without close family ties or in dysfunctional family units, with roommates with limited personal interaction, not dating offline, no offline friends), apart from situational contact (e.g., with store clerks when purchasing food, and perhaps at work) and being physically present with their i-tech devices on beaches, at bus stops, or in line at the grocery store, some people's lives are now lived entirely online. They have no offline relationships!

This indeed has the properties of futuristic sci-fi! A culture or subculture that functions without any, or at best extremely limited, non-digitally mediated human interaction, and no (human) touch…

Scientific Corner: A subsequent examination of responses on the IAT revealed that uniformly individuals who were not in partnerships or interactive cohabitation responded "does not apply" to the five questions on Dr. Young's test designed to evaluate "interference with family relationships." Given that, in the test, the classification of "does not apply" is scored as zero in a 0 to 5 sum system (this is where you add up all the numbers to calculate severity; the higher the number, the more severe), scores for these single people would never be high enough to score as problematic use. At best, all these individuals would come up with a designation of mild Internet addiction. Ironic indeed. (The questions that were systematically affected were: 3, 5, 9, 13, and 18 (see Young, 1998, 2011). Here I introduce an argument that the model becomes three dimensional (see ***Scientific Corner*** above for dimensions). Alternately, it can be argued that the fourth dimension is or has become the Internet. The selection of the category "does not apply/non applicable" (Young, 1998, 2011) can either speak to a reduced level of interference in real-life interpersonal relationships or, in contrast, it speaks to the absolute nonexistence of real-life interpersonal relationships due to total immersion in the technology. In the case of my study, it would appear to be the latter. There is now a profile of adult Internet user who has disengaged from offline life to such an extent that the IAT, as currently scored, may no longer be applied as an accurate measure of severity of Internet Addiction. At its extreme, an individual who is physically or socially isolated from family, does not have offline friends, is not partnered or dating, is not attending school, and is unemployed will potentially respond "does not apply" to all questions that are designed to evaluate disruption to education, to work, and to existing real-life interpersonal relationships. In sum, it is possible that individuals with the lowest scores may also be those most severely affected.

We may already be there...Virtual reality and robots are a thriving area of research and development. We are developing interactive mini-robots for children as well as very adult robots, dolls, and toys designed exclusively for sexual purpose. There is a whole industry involved in the development of what is now called sexnology, technology that permits the illusion of touch of real distal people via screens or of fantasy characters, again via screens and body gear. In essence, there is great interest in the last frontier of i-tech, the mimicking of human relationships including touch.

What Really Is i-Addiction and Who Defines It?

So is withdrawing from physical space with physical humans to i-tech and an exclusively i-mediated world truly an addiction? Or is the notion of i-addiction entirely framed by digital immigrants (such as myself) who cannot relate to the behavior, people who openly admit we fear living in an impersonal world depicted by our

> Is this behavior merely an anomaly that will remain a lifestyle for a select group, or is it a foreshadowing of things to come?

adolescent sci-fi (e.g., *Blade Runner*, and later the *Total Recall* series)? Is this behavior merely an anomaly that will remain a lifestyle for a select group, or is it a foreshadowing of things to come?

Here again I bow to definitions and multiple realities. Addiction by definition is the relentless pursuit of something that harms: a dysfunction in brain circuitry that results in the biological, psychological, spiritual, and social traits associated with maladaptive pursuit and usage (paraphrased from ASAM, 2011) So who are supposed i-addicts harming and where is the dysfunction?

The young and the old who cross my clinical floor are clearly harming themselves and their families. They are suffering from behavioral and conduct disorders, learning disabilities, emotional deregulation (predominantly depression and anxiety, intimacy disorders, and sexual dysfunction). For youth, the classification of failure to thrive also has a gross impact on others: first, direct family, and thereafter the rest of society. These "non-participants" who withdraw to i-tech are directly hostaging family with their choice to disconnect from the real world per se. They seek empathy for depression or anxiety yet want autonomy to be online. They often use emotional blackmail, demanding to be emotionally and financially supported including being fed, sheltered, clothed, and yes supplied with i-tech devices and the service contracts on which they function. When family withdraws from the role, larger society picks up the tab through social services (typically disability services or welfare).

But what about those who support themselves: those who are gainfully employed, tax-paying, law-abiding citizens, who merely prefer to live all possible aspects of their lives online? Who are they harming: arguably no one. Or are they?

And here we have the second layer of truth: fear. As with the international students presented in the introduction, whose behavior foreshadowed digital interface being the primary method of communication for youth, many of us now fear that i-tech will replace human interface, all human interface. And it terrifies us.

Unlike the standard language and cultural issues that divide generations, immigrants and natives, or otherwise pre-settled peoples of different cultures and all walks of life, i-tech is threatening our notions of humanity. And the science appears to be supporting this.

We are facing much more than actual or perceived threats on language, tradition, religion, politics, or even philosophy. We are facing threats on emotional availability, sensitivity, and perception; memory, processing, learning, and intelligence; creativity, artistry, and innovation; arousal, desensitization, disinhibition, and reactivity; and finally, development, attachment, and pair bonding that fundamentally propagate our species.

We are further facing sex technology (sexnology) including functional robotic equipment and dolls; parenting technology AKA babysitting games and toys; and friendship technology, including sites, programs, and toys that mimic people. We have the first groups of individuals explicitly choosing to engage hours upon hours with technology and behind screens instead of with each other in person or in body.

As we see billions upon billions spent on research and development and millions upon millions of people choosing to purchase and engage with the products produced, some of us are asking what is the critical mass, what is the tipping point, that will change global culture, all of society as we know it, and yes, our notions of humanity itself.

CHAPTER FOURTEEN

Final Thoughts

Turn Off the Bells

I would like to conclude with yet another little personal story. It was Christmas time at least thirty-odd years ago. I was a young teenager at the time, waiting patiently in line with my grandmother at a local department store. The line was long, and the store was understaffed. In fact there was only one clerk behind the counter trying to process a line of at least twenty of us eager to pay for our merchandise and go home to our festivities. What was remarkable, however, was not the speed at which or which not the clerk was processing us all, nor the stores lack of oversight in holiday staffing, but that every time the counter phone rang the clerk would abandon the client she was serving and indirectly all of us present. She would answer the phone and tend to whatever the person on the other end of it needed. A price check, a return policy, store hours, whatever. Despite the length of the line, our obvious disappointment, the huffing, the rolling of eyes, direct verbalizations or other explicit expression of resentment of those of us in line, that we had been waiting sequentially, nor even the fact that we, the present, all were explicitly going to purchase and pay for merchandise bringing the store instant profit, the ring of the phone superseded us all.

Arguably, such response to sounds or calls is not limited to my childhood observations. Long long before telephones and i-tech, we responded to such sounds this way: dinner bells, school bells, church bells, dropping other including personal interaction to tend to, or follow the message sent by, said bell. Which makes one wonder: Are we wired this way? Are we wired to respond to sounds, buttons, or calls? Have we just finally evolved into an era where the frequency of these calls, bells, or sounds is problematic? Again, do accessibility and "moreness" have us unilaterally falling prey to bells and tones as moths to the flame?

If anyone cares to look it up, there was much research for many years on what we referred to as the P3, P300 or ERP brainwave (*event related potential*), a reactive brainwave that distinctly indicated startle, or differentiated things unusual from the usual in the visual, olfactory, or auditory field (e.g., seeing a snake, an unusual or out-of-context sound or smell). The wave is indicative that we will react. This response is hardwired in us for safety, for action, or for alertness to our environment. Is it all as simple as the sounds of i-tech do this to us, and then we get sucked in by our own process waiting, wanting the instant arousal, the stimulus of this little wave, this little reaction?

What is evident is there is just something bewitching about the buzz, the ring, and now the endless possibility for more: instant accessibility both in content and material, attainable. Like Pavlov's dog we have conditioned ourselves to salivate to the bell, like lab rats we push and push on the lever for the food pellet of pleasure, of intrigue, of more. What we have forgotten to ask is what is happening to our brains in this great experiment of life on i-tech.

From my perspective, the whole phenomenon of our current malcontent has to do with too much. And the Internet and i-tech are collectively the supreme tools, the icing on the cake, of the massive convergence of too much more. Too much food, hence obesity. Too much product, combined with too much credit, hence mass consumerism and focus on objects as opposed to people, with the byproduct of too much debt. Too much access to medical information, hence cyberchondria. Too many shows available, hence series binging. Too much access and availability of pornography, hence the loss of intimacy. Too many options for partners on Internet dating, hence the loss of satisfaction and pair bonding. Too many Facebook friends, hence truly close to no one. Too much information leading to the consumption of trivia as opposed to the acquisition and assimilation of knowledge.

It's just too much: hence we are unraveling, like robots with overloaded circuits when they can no longer assimilate or manage all the data. We are breaking down in anxiety and depression due to never being satiated, never satisfied...There is always more! But how much more can we handle and remain ourselves: remain human?

So What to Do?

So now that we have gone around the world in exploring the dynamics of structured and unstructured learning; organized and unorganized play; the role of caregivers in socio-emotional development, and pathology with extra emphasis on anxiety, failed attachment, restriction and over-structure, learning disabilities, communication, sexuality and the new online and only online world, what do we do about it?

If this is the way you want to live your life, do. Who am I, or any other psychologist, philosopher, MD, or neurologist to pontificate or tell you otherwise? That said, the whole purpose of this book is to raise awareness, to be conscious of the choices we make and their global socio-emotional effect on an entire culture: on human culture not just on self.

But for those of you who have children, want them, or are in any professional or charitable capacity that is of direct influence (e.g., educator, MD, psychologist, psychiatrist, or coach), I think we can not quite yet abdicate our roles vis-à-vis social responsibility in this era of mass shifting.

If I did not see the undeniable connection with socio-sexual-emotional deregulation, the reduction or hijacking of innovation and creative process, learning disabilities, depression, and anxiety, anxiety, so much anxiety: an epidemic of hyper-arousal...if I did not directly see this both in society and now also in the brain, I would retire my keyboard and, as Prensky says, work on correcting my Digital Immigrant accent, let go of the hang-ups my generation tends to hold on to, and let the digital natives do what's best, for them and perhaps us too.

But I don't quite see it so black and white. Hence, like the frontpiece of this book and Janus the Roman God of passages, doorways, gates, beginnings, and transitions depicted, I believe we owe it to ourselves to keep one face, one mind, firmly fixed on the past while the other mind bravely looks forward, embracing change.

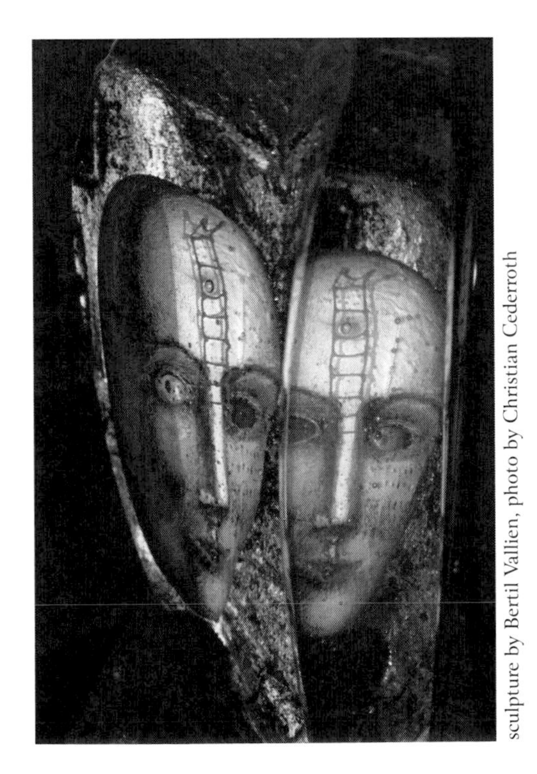

sculpture by Bertil Vallien, photo by Christian Cederroth

Epilogue

Part A. Action Plan: Countering Social Apathy

If you like the role of i-tech in your personal and professional world, embrace it. If you don't like it and what it is doing to your world, disengage. Not in everything, not always, but return to using it wisely as a tool, the wonderful, magnificent, and extremely efficient tool and delivery system that it is. But let's not let this tool, this system, rule us, regulate us (or should I say, deregulate us).

1. Key in this is the setting of boundaries; one I have, for example, is that I do not reply to work emails past a specific hour or on weekends. I may (not so secretly) write them but I very rarely send them until "office hours." My colleagues know this; my clients know this. Hence no one is desperately waiting for my input on an issue or a response. As a result, I am not so anxious, always "on call," and can, and do, often relax, free of work duties for an evening, a day, and on occasion, a week or two!

2. Second, and perhaps most important of all, let's all take

back play! Sure, play with i-tech but let's also play with our children, with our partners, with our friends. Let's get back to our dinner parties, our bedrooms, our coffee shops, our (i)books, our soccer and baseball games, our toys, our parks, fields, woods, gardens, and lakes and occasionally leave the digital devices behind. Turn them off completely for an evening or at very least an hour or two. Let's take back painting, drawing, board games and comedy clubs, observation, pondering, creativity, and touch. Let's take back some non-tech life!

To Do List

- Take back play and don't get caught in the organization and the capitalism of it all.
- Remove elitism from arts and sports.
- Fight like hell to have sport, music, and art reintroduced in schools during the curriculum. (Children will find ample structure under the guidance of teachers and competition between schools and districts.)
- Bring back hobbies where, by definition, being good or bad at them is irrelevant! (Again be attentive to those that are completely commercially driven. A child does not need a $50.00 monthly budget at a craft store for the "appropriate" stickers and beads, and corner protectors of scrapbooking. Collage and papier-mâché are relatively cost-free (*and* require significantly more creativity)!
- Fight like hell to have classroom size reduced, so that if a little one, or two, go "off task" it is not a critical issue for classroom management.
- Fight like hell to have fields and parks built and maintained,

and yes, kept interesting. (Don't sue if your children hurt themselves having fun.)

- Don't get caught in "getting what you pay for" in early childhood education. (Yes childcare is expensive; but there is no extra value in your five-year-old coming home having learned that red is the color of the toy box, fire engines, and sometimes apples. He or she will figure all that out on their own anyway when the time is right. There is value in your child coming home with a sleepy smile from running around all day and red paint under her or his fingernails.)
- In formal education ensure that the integration of technologies serves a true educational purpose, and is not merely introduced because of novelty, convenience, or vested external interests.
- Get back to your beds as opposed to your computers together. Snuggle, touch and be touched by people, by each other.
- Play! Play with your children, your partners, your friends, your pets and any and all non-tech objects around you.

Part B. Unique Kids and Direction Versus Correction

As hinted to earlier, part of the problem with kids is actually adults' own over-arousal and related higher stress levels. Being "stressed out," we are less tolerant, less accepting of children's natural behavior. As fallout we have lost sight of the fact that children, just like adults, come in different forms with different personalities. Many children, by nature of just being children, are what I affectionately call wiggly pigglies, and some, purely by their own nature, extremely so.

These busy children, unless overtly engaged, squirm, move, find things and touch them, take their shoes on and off...essentially they find things to do to entertain themselves in absence of other stimulation or when in otherwise "uninteresting" environments. In contrast to busy kids, there are also those whom I refer to as kinetic kids: these are kids that simply must move. For these select children restricting movement is akin to pain; without movement or some form of self-stimulation, life is torture. This again is not necessarily ADHD; it is just the miniature version of a very kinetic individual, one with great athletic and innovative promise. Many of us fit the profile as children; most of us over time have just learned to regulate our movement in age-appropriate and socially appropriate manners. Some would say we "grow out of ADHD."

In my professional opinion, we did not grow out of anything; we simply grew out of childhood and child-like expression of movement, which just happens to be particularly annoying to some conservative sectors and some stressed-out or overworked adults. Period! Again not new: across cultures, generations, and even eras before us, we had tools or inclusive mechanisms that catered to kinetic people. In most of Arabia, some of Persia, and Southern Europe, there was the pocket or finger stone, in Greece there was the movable fish, in many Asian and European cultures there were hand-held beads or beaded bracelets. The Catholic Church even figured it out with the rosary, as did other religions with prayer beads and wheels; you can't ask people to pray for hours on end without some tactile stimulation or for that matter physical ritual.

We need to let go of the current medical misconception that the need for movement or otherwise kinetic stimulation is for kids, is exclusive to boys, and is undesirable. Look at early female parlor activities in the most conservative of times, such as needlework or embroidery in the Victorian era. Nowadays, how many pairs of knitted pink booties, pot holders, or toilet paper covers do we need? Surely not as many as produced: elderly women need kinetic stimulation too and many find it through the knitting, the crocheting of anything. Apart from nicotine addiction, why was smoking and tobacco chewing so popular over the centuries...and gum, the porch swing, the rocking chair. The list goes on.

We need to move. Hours and hours at our desks in classrooms or offices, sitting in chairs at movies or on sofas with our i-tech devices, do us no good. We need to move as it is healthy for us, for our whole biological system. Early on we noted how television watching, or rather the sedentary action that came with watching, was not only associated with obesity but with learning disabilities, not for all the issues regarding content and process aforementioned, but because it deregulated the dopamine system, which again regulates attention and all executive function.[232] Today it is any i-device or computer. They appear to be affecting the same dopaminergic systems but they are also affecting our metabolism via our hormones directly governing weight gain and sleep cycles. If you are in front of a screen at night, your body will not produce melatonin; this will deregulate general arousal states but so too sleep cycles and circadian rhythm.[233] In sum you will not be regulated in your natural sleep/wake, relaxed/arousal cycles for which we are all biologically designed in cohesion with dark and light, the sun and moon.

Back to children, the key to what I refer to as busy and kinetic children is not to suppress. As mentioned previously, it is torture. In the case of school, if successful in repression, the child will be entirely focused on not moving as opposed to on the lesson; it is a lose-lose situation for learning. With such children, I coach parents to in turn coach their children to find socially acceptable age-appropriate subtle kinetic activities. And apart from stretch breaks under the guise of being a teacher's assistant (passing out papers, plugging in equipment, or sharpening pencils), not to pander, you want your child to adapt to their environment and not have the environment adapt to them (*many special adaptations are potentially a recipe for failure, identification with disability, and future entitlement for adaptations at college and work thereafter*). As such, no special wiggle seats, or stress balls that can become wonderful projectiles: just something subtle the child can fiddle with, that can't be dropped, can't be thrown, can't be overtly played with, does not have negative social stigma (like hair twirling or any item with chewing capacity), and does not make noise as the child pays attention. Essentially something that does not affect classroom management or the child's own ability to focus. The fact is, for many kinetic people, stimming helps with focus. This is an opportunity for children to learn what helps and to thereafter be responsible for the maintenance of their own attention.

Out of school, engage in what I refer to as thrill and chill activities: activities where the brain and body become aroused and then fatigue together – trampoline, pogo sticks, skateboards, biking, skipping.

So why am I ending this book, spending so much time describing, and then coaching, on what to do with busy or kinetic children? Because these are precisely the children most seriously at risk. Such highly wired brains seek stimulation and will find it. Such brains will be drawn to i-tech, become mesmerized by it. Thereafter, if not mediated, the technology will entrain the need for more arousal as opposed to less.

And, because these exact children can become the most wonderful of adults...

What Busy Brains and Bodies Can Grow Up to Be

Kinetic children are busy children; no surprise, they grow up to be busy adults. They make great athletes, presenters, sales, and front people precisely because of this "energy." They also make great entrepreneurs. As adults we like these people; we are drawn to them for their magnetism. This vibrant energy, once corralled or harnessed toward good, can lead to great success.

I was once attending a meeting of very successful entrepreneurs and business people, and I mean very. It was a long meeting; three and a half hours in fact. As everyone spoke, everyone listened, attentively, fully engaged. But what I also noticed was everyone, every single individual around the table, was also doing something else. There was some sort of kinetic expression; some sort of stimming. One was playing with a pen, another a napkin, one was fingering glasses, and yes one was even doodling. But I guarantee you, everyone was fully present, attentive. These are what busy minds grow into – with the proper direction not correction, and certainly not suppression.

Busy brained people remain mentally and often kinetically engaged with their environments. And, just like children, such adults are at higher risk for abuse or overuse of i-tech. As busy brains always need and want something to do, they will turn to i-devices; check phones or other portable i-devices in meetings or immediately upon breaks, not because they are missing anything critical at home or business, just because it is the twenty-first century version of stimming.

Fifteen years ago during breaks people would turn to each other, little side conversations could and would spark; now too, but less. The first reaction now, for most, is to check their i-tech devices, to start side conversations with those distal or tend to the messages received. I am not saying people would not excuse themselves earlier, make phone calls, check in, but not with such frequency, or perceived urgency or expectation, and certainly not to the exclusion of individuals actually physically present. This is the issue: it is not i-tech or no i-tech. It is the i-tech override.

It is very easy to polarize the issues with mannerisms, habits, attitudes, and disdain expressed by digital immigrants versus digital natives on the way things should be. Other divides are between those with vested versus non-vested interests, including those working in clinical practice versus those with a pulse on the general population. When we over-engage in such arguments, I fear we are all missing the point.

It is very easy to polarize the issues with mannerisms, habits, attitudes, and disdain expressed by digital immigrants versus digital natives on the way things should be.

We are undeniably in a mass societal

shift, a mass experiment of sorts with no idea of the outcome. As such, I believe we owe it to ourselves, and the generations still under our care, to keep our eyes wide open: to keep looking, keep examining, keep questioning, and be equally open to change and the potential of the future as to the wisdom of the past. Until we have a better idea of where we are going, and at what cost or advantage, let's keep a little of what used to keep us happy and, perhaps more importantly, more connected.

Appendix

Reliability of the Data Set

Intraclass Correlation Coefficient

		95% Confidence Interval		*F Test with True Value 0*			
Measures	**Intraclass Correlation[a]**	**Lower Bound**	**Upper Bound**	**Value**	**df1**	**df2**	**Sig**
Single	.999[b]	.999	.999	2025.627	125	125	·.001
Average	.999[c]	.999	1.000	2025.627	125	125	·.001

Note. Two-way mixed effects model where people effects are random and measures effects are fixed.

[a]Type A intraclass correlation coefficients using an absolute agreement definition.

[b]The estimator is the same, whether the interaction effect is present or not.

[c]This estimate is computed assuming the interaction effect is absent, because it is not estimable otherwise.

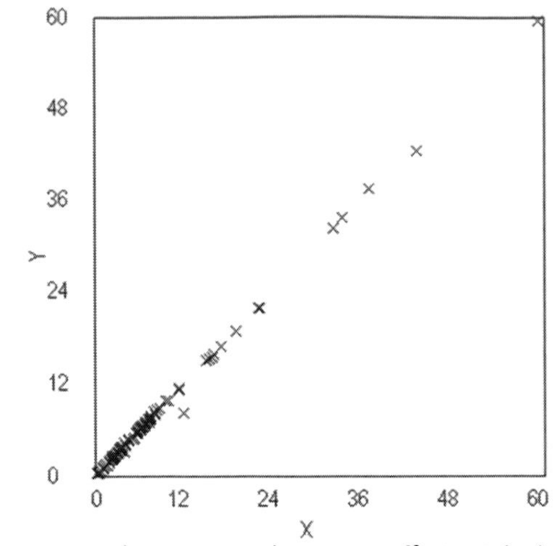

Sample concordance correlation coefficient (ρc) = 0.9989
Figure 1. Reliability of data set: concordance results.

Endnotes

1 Chou, C., Condron, L., & Belland, J.C. (2005). A review of the research on IA. *Educational Psychology Review, 17*(4), 363–388.

2 Young, K.S. (1998). IA: The emergence of a new clinical disorder. *CyberPsychology and Behavior, 1*(3), 237–244.

3 Griffiths, M. (1998). IA: Does it really exist? In J. Gackenbach (Ed.), *Psychology and the Internet: Intrapersonal, interpersonal, and transpersonal implications* (pp. 61–75). New York, NY: Academic Press.

4 Chou, C., Chou, J., & Tran, T.T. (1999). An exploratory study of IA, usage and communication pleasure: The Taiwanese case. *International Journal of Education and Communication, 5*(1), 47–64.

5 Kandell, J.J. (1998). IA on campus: The vulnerability of college students. *CyberPsychology and Behavior, 1*(1), 11–17.

6 Orzack, M.H. (1999). Computer addiction: Is it real or virtual? *Harvard Mental Health Letter, 15*(7), 8.

7 Young, K.S. (1996). IA: The emergence of a new clinical disorder. *CyberPsychology and Behavior, 1*(3), 237–244.

8 Prensky, M. (2001). Digital Natives, Digital Immigrants, Part One. *On the Horizon, 9*(5), 1–6.

9 Not to be confused with the six generations: Greatest, Silent, Baby Boomer, and Gens X, Y, and Z. See Weiss, R. & Schneider, J. (2014). *Closer Together, Further Apart*. Carefree, Arizona: Gentle Path Press.

10 Caplan, S.E., & High, A.C. (2011). Online social interaction, psychological well-being, and problematic Internet use. In K.S. Young, & C.N.

Nabuco de Abreu (Eds.), *Internet Addiction* (pp. 35–54). Hoboken, NJ: John Wiley & Sons.

11 Greenfield, D.N. (1999). Psychological characteristics of compulsive Internet use: A preliminary analysis. *CyberPsychology and Behavior, 8*(5), 403–412.

12 Young, K. S. (1998). *Caught in the net: How to recognise the signs of Internet addiction and a winning strategy for recovery.* NY, NY: John Wiley & Sons.

13 Rosen, L (2012). iDisorder. New York, NY: Palgrave.

14 Shaffer, H.J. (1996). Understanding the means and objects of addiction: Technology, the Internet and gambling. *Journal of Gambling Studies, 12*(4), 461–469.

15 Sigman, A. (2005). *Remotely controlled*. London, UK: Random House.

16 Swingle, M. (2013). *Electroencephalographic (EEG) brainmap patterns in a clinical sample of adults diagnosed with an Internet addiction*. PhD Dissertation. Fielding Graduate University.

17 Ibid.

18 Jang, K.L. (2005). *The behavioral genetics of psychopathology.* Mahwah, NJ: Lawrence Erlbaum.

19 Kendler, S.K., & Prescott, C.A. (2006). *Genes, environment, and psychopathology*. New York, NY: Guilford Press.

20 Rutter, M. (2006). *Genes and behavior: Nature-nurture interplay explained*. Malden, MA: Blackwell.

21 Rutter, M. (Ed.). (2008). *Genetic effects on environmental vulnerability*. Chichester, UK: Wiley & Sons

22 Sroufe, L.A., Egeland, B., Carlson, A., & Collins, W.A. (2005). *The development of the person*. New York, NY: Guilford Press.

23 Beard, K.W. (2008). IA in children and adolescents. In C.B. Yarnall (Ed.), *Computer science research trends* (pp. 59–70). Hauppauge, NY: Nova Scotia.

24 Jang, K.S., Hwang, S.Y., & Choi, J.Y. (2008). IA and psychiatric symptoms among Korean adolescents. *Journal of School Health, 78*(3), 165–171.

25 Young, K.S., & Nabuco de Abreu, C. N. (Eds.). (2011). *Internet addiction.* Hoboken, NJ: John Wiley & Sons.)

26 Ha, J.H., Yoo, H.J., Cho, I., Chin, B., Shin, D., & Kim, J.H. (2006). Psychiatric comorbidity assessed in Korean children and adolescents who screen positive for IA. *Journal of Clinical Psychiatry, 67,* 821–826.

27 Kim, K.H., Ryu, E.J., Chon, M.Y., Yeun, E.J., Choi, S.Y., & Seo, J.S. (2006). IA in Korean adolescents and its relation to depression and suicidal ideation: A questionnaire survey. *International Journal of Nursing Studies, 43*(2) 185–192.

28 Lin, S.J., & Tsai, C.C. (2002). Sensation seeking and Internet dependence of Taiwanese high school adolescents. *Computers in Human Behavior, 18*, 411–426.

29 Ryu, E., Choi, K.S., Seo, J.S, & Nam, B.W. (2004). The relationship of IA, depression, and suicidal ideation in adolescents. *Journal of Korean Academy of Nursing, 34*(1), 102–110.

30 Caplan, S.E., & High, A.C. (2011). Online social interaction, psychological well-being, and problematic Internet use. In K.S. Young, & C.N. Nabuco de Abreu, (Eds.), *Internet addiction* (pp. 35–54). Hoboken, NJ: John Wiley & Sons.

31 Beard, K.W. (2008). IA in children and adolescents. In C.B. Yarnall (Ed.), *Computer science research trends* (pp. 59–70). Hauppauge, NY: Nova Scotia.

32 Ha, J.H., Yoo, H.J., Cho, I., Chin, B., Shin, D., & Kim, J.H. (2006). Psychiatric comorbidity assessed in Korean children and adolescents who screen positive for IA. *Journal of Clinical Psychiatry, 67*, 821–826.

33 Jang, K.S., Hwang, S.Y., & Choi, J.Y. (2008). IA and psychiatric symptoms among Korean adolescents. *Journal of School Health, 78*(3), 165–171.

34 Kim, K.H., Ryu, E.J., Chon, M.Y., Yeun, E.J., Choi, S.Y., & Seo, J.S. (2006). IA in Korean adolescents and its relation to depression and suicidal ideation: A questionnaire survey. *International Journal of Nursing Studies, 43*(2) 185–192.

35 Lin, S.J., & Tsai, C.C. (2002). Sensation seeking and Internet dependence of Taiwanese high school adolescents. *Computers in Human Behavior, 18*, 411–426.

36 Ryu, E., Choi, K.S., Seo, J.S, & Nam, B.W. (2004). The relationship of IA, depression, and suicidal ideation in adolescents. *Journal of Korean Academy of Nursing, 34*(1), 102–110.

37 Young, K.S., & Nabuco de Abreu, C. N. (Eds.). (2011). *Internet addiction*. Hoboken, NJ: John Wiley & Sons.

38 Swingle, M. (2013). *Electroencephalographic (EEG) brainmap patterns in a clinical sample of adults diagnosed with an Internet addiction*. PhD Dissertation. Fielding Graduate University.

39 Caplan, S.E., & High, A.C. (2011). Online social interaction, psychological well-being, and problematic Internet use. In K.S. Young, & C.N. Nabuco de Abreu, (Eds.), *Internet addiction* (pp. 35–54). Hoboken, NJ: John Wiley & Sons)

40 Caplan, S.E. (2010). Theory and measurement of generalized problematic Internet use. *CyberPsychology and Behavior, 10*, 234–241.

41 Ibid.

42 Caplan, S.E. (2003). Preference for online social interaction: A theory

of problematic Internet use and psychosocial well-being. *Communication Research, 30*, 625–648.

43 Caplan, S.E. (2005). A social skill account of problematic Internet use. *Journal of Communication, 55*, 721–736.

44 [44] Erwin, B.A., Turk, C.L., Heimberg, R.G., Fresco, D.M., & Hantula, D.A. (2004). The Internet: Home to a severe population of individuals with social anxiety disorder? *Anxiety Disorders, 18*, 629–646.

45 Davis, R.A., Flett, G.L., & Besser, A. (2002). Validation of a new scale for measuring problematic Internet use: Implications for pre-employment screening. *CyberPsychology and Behavior, 5*, 331–345.

46 High, A., & Caplan, S.E. (2009). Social anxiety and computer-mediated communications during initial interactions: Implications for the hyperpersonal perspective. *Computers in Human Behavior, 25*, 475–482.

47 Morahan-Martin, J., & Schumacher, P. (2003). Loneliness and social uses of the Internet. *Computers in Human Behavior, 19*, 659–671.

48 Swingle, P. (2008). *Biofeedback for the brain.* Piscataway, NJ: Rutgers University Press.

49 Bruder, G.E., Fong, R., Tenke, C.E., Leite, P., Towey, J.P., Stewart, J.E., McGrath, P.J., & Quitkin, F.M. (1997). Regional brain asymmetries in major depression with or without anxiety disorder: A quantitative electroencephalographic study. *Biological Psychiatry, 41*, 939–948.

50 Henriques, J.B., & Davidson, R.J. (1990). Regional brain electrical asymmetries discriminate between previously depressed and health control subject. *Journal of Abnormal Psychology, 99*, 22–31.

51 Henriques, J.B., & Davidson, R.J. (1991). Left frontal hypoactivation in depression. *Journal of Abnormal Psychology, 100*, 534–45.

52 Swingle, P. (2008). *Biofeedback for the brain.* Piscataway, NJ: Rutgers University Press.

53 Young, K.S., & Nabuco de Abreu, C. N. (Eds.). (2011). *Internet addiction.* Hoboken, NJ: John Wiley & Sons.

54 Young, K.S., & Rodgers, R.C. (1998). The relationship between depression and Internet Addiction. *Cyber Psychology and Behavior, 1*(1), 25–28.

55 Caplan, S.E., & High, A.C. (2011). Online social interaction, psychological well-being, and problematic Internet use. In K.S. Young, & C.N. Nabuco de Abreu, (Eds.), *Internet addiction* (pp. 35–54). Hoboken, NJ: John Wiley & Sons.

56 Ha, J.H., Yoo, H.J., Cho, I., Chin, B., Shin, D., & Kim, J.H. (2006). Psychiatric comorbidity assessed in Korean children and adolescents who screen positive for IA. *Journal of Clinical Psychiatry, 67,* 821–826.

57 Young, K.S., & Nabuco de Abreu, C. N. (Eds.). (2011). *Internet addiction.* Hoboken, NJ: John Wiley & Sons.

58 Caplan, S.E., Williams, D., & Lee, N. (2009). Problematic Internet use and psychosocial well-being among MMO players. *Computers in Human Behavior, 25*(6), 1312–1319.

59 Bostwick, J.M., & Bucci, J.A. (2008). Internet sex addiction treated with naltrexone. *Mayo Clinic Proceedings, 83*(2), 226–230.

60 Dell'Osso, B., Hadley, S., Allen, A., Baker, B., Chaplin, W.F., & Hollander, E. (2008). Escitalopram in the treatment of impulsive-compulsive Internet usage disorder: An open-label trial followed by a double-blind discontinuation phase. *Journal of Clinical Psychiatry, 69*(3), 452–456.

61 Raymond, N.C., Coleman, E., & Miner, M.H. (2003). Psychiatric comorbidity and compulsive/impulsive traits in compulsive sexual behavior. *Comprehensive Psychiatry, 44,* 370-380.

62 Kafka, M. (2000). Psychopharmacological treatments for nonparaphilic compulsive sexual behaviors. *CNS Spectrums, 5,* 49-59.

63 Karim, R. (2009). Cutting edge pharmacology for sex addiction: How do the meds work? A presentation for the Society for the Advancement of Sexual Health, San Diego, CA.

64 Raymond, N.C., Grant, J.E., Kim, S.W., & Coleman, E. (2002). Treating compulsive sexual behavior with naltrexone and serotonin reuptake inhibitors: Two case studies. *International Clinical Psychopharmacology,* 17, 201-205.

65 Fontenelle, L.F., Oostermeijer, S., Harrison, B.J., Pantelis, C., & Yucel, M. (2011). Obsessive-Compulsive Disorder, Impulse Control Disorders and drug addiction. *Drugs, 7*(7), 827-840.).

66 Ibid.

67 Pies, R. (2009). Should DSM-V designate "Internet Addiction" a mental disorder? *Psychiatry, 6*(2), 31–37.

68 te Wildt, B.T., Putzig, I., Drews, M., Lampen-Imkamp, S., Zedler, M., Weise, B., Dillo, W., & Ohlmeier, M.D. (2010). Pathological Internet use and psychiatric disorders: A cross-sectional study on psychiatric phenomenology and clinical relevance of Internet dependency. *The European Journal of Psychiatry, 24*(3). Retrieved from http://dx.doi.org

69 Dell'Osso, B., Hadley, S., Allen, A., Baker, B., Chaplin, W.F., & Hollander, E. (2008). Escitalopram in the treatment of impulsive-compulsive Internet usage disorder: An open-label trial followed by a double-blind discontinuation phase. *Journal of Clinical Psychiatry, 69*(3), 452–456.

70 Shapira, N.A., Goldsmith, T.D., Keck, P.E., Kohosia, U.M., & McElroy,

S.L. (2000). Psychiatric features of individuals with problematic Internet use. *Journal of Affective Disorders, 57*, 267–272.

71 Black, D.W., Belsare, G., & Schlosser, S. (1999). Clinical features, psychiatric co-morbidity, and health-related quality of life in persons reporting compulsive computer use behavior. *Journal of Clinical Psychiatry, 60*(12), 839–844.

72 Bernardi, S., & Palanti, S. (2008). Internet Addiction: A descriptive clinical study focusing on co-morbidities and dissociative symptoms. *Comprehensive Psychiatry, 50*(6), 510–516.

73 Caplan, S.E., Williams, D., & Lee, N. (2009). Problematic Internet use and psychosocial well-being among MMO players. *Computers in Human Behavior, 25*(6), 1312–1319.

74 Weiss, R. & Schneider, J. (2014). *Closer Together, Further Apart*. Carefree, Arizona: Gentle Path Press.

75 Small, G. & Vorgan, G. (2008). Your brain is evolving right now. In *The Digital Divide*. M. Bauerlein (Ed.) London, UK: Penguin Books.

76 Newfeld, G., & Mate, G. (2004). *Hold on to your kids*. Toronto, Canada: Random House.

77 Porges, S. (2011). *The polyvagal theory: Neurophysiologial foundations of emotions, attachment, communication, and self-regulation.* New York: W. W. Norton & Company.

78 Block, J.J. (2008). Issues for DSM-V: IA. *American Journal of Psychiatry, 165*, 306–307.

79 Cooney, G.M., & Morris, J. (2009). Time to start taking an Internet history? *The British Journal of Psychiatry, 194,* 185.

80 Kim, K.H., Ryu, E.J., Chon, M.Y., Yeun, E.J., Choi, S.Y., & Seo, J.S. (2006). IA in Korean adolescents and its relation to depression and suicidal ideation: A questionnaire survey. *International Journal of Nursing Studies, 43*(2) 185–192.

81 Ko, C.H., Yen, J.Y., Chen, C.S., Yeh, Y.C., & Yen, C.F. (2009). Predictive values of psychiatric symptoms for Internet addiction in adolescents. *Archives of Pediatric Adolescent Medicine, 163*(10), 937–943.

82 Cooney, G.M., & Morris, J. (2009). Time to start taking an Internet history? *The British Journal of Psychiatry, 194,* 185.

83 Gentile, D. A. (2009). Pathological video game use among youth 8–18: A national study. Psychological Science, 20, 594–602.

84 Hammond, C., & Gunkelman, J. (2001). *The art of artifacting.* McLean, VA: Society for Neuronal Regulation.

85 Thatcher, R.W., & Lubar, J. F., (2009). History of the scientific standards of QEEG normative databases. In T.H. Budzynski, H.G. Budzynski,

J.R. Evans, & A. Abarnel (Eds.), *Quantitative EEG and neurofeedback* (pp. 29–59). San Diego, CA: Academic Press.

86 Swingle, P. (2008). *Biofeedback for the brain.* Piscataway, NJ: Rutgers University Press.

87 Hartmann, T. (1999). Whose order is being disordered by AD/HD? *Tikkun, 14,* 17–21.

88 Hartmann, T. (2003). *The Edison gene*. Rochester, Vermont: Park Street Press.

89 Mathewson, K, E, Basak, C, Maclin, E.L., Boot, W.R., Kramer, A.F., Fabiani, M., & Gratton, G. (2012). Different slopes for different folks: Alpha and delta EEG power predict subsequent video game learning rate and improvements in cognitive control tasks. *Psychophysiology*, 49 (12), 1558–1570.

90 Boot, W.R., Blakely, D.P. and Simons, D.J. (2011) Do Action Video Games Improve Perception and Cognition? *Frontiers in Psychology*, 2011; DOI: 10.3389/fpsyg.2011.00226

91 Jay Pratt et al.(2014). The effect of action video game playing on sensorimotor learning: Evidence from a movement tracking task. *Human Movement Science*. DOI: 10.1016/j.humov.2014.09.004

92 Parish-Morris, J., Mahajan, N., Hirsh-Pasek, K., Michnick Golinkoff, R., & Fuller Colllins, M. (2013). Once Upon a Time: Parent–Child Dialogue and Storybook Reading in the Electronic Era. *Mind, Brain, and Education*, *7* (3), 200–211.

93 Swingle, P. (2008). *Biofeedback for the brain.* Piscataway, NJ: Rutgers University Press.

94 Thomas, M. (2008). On vines and minds. *The Psychologist, 21*(5), 378–381.

95 Weinstein, A.M. (2010). Computer and game addiction: A comparison between game users and non game users. *The American Journal of Drug and Alcohol Abuse, 36*(5), 268–276.

96 Ko, C.H., Liu, G.C., Hsiao, S., Yen, J.Y., Yang, M.J., Lin, W.C., Yen, C.F, & Chen, C.S. (2009). Brain activities associated with gaming urge of online gaming addiction. *Journal of Psychiatric Research, 43*, 739-747.

97 Han, D.H., Bolo, N., Daniels, M.A., Arenella, L., Lyoo, K., & Renshaw, P.F. (2011). Brain activity and desire for Internet video game play. *Comprehensive Psychiatry, 52*, 88-95.

98 Kalivas, P.W., & Volkow, N.D. (2005). The neural basis of addiction: A pathology of motivation and choice. *American Journal of Psychiatry, 162*, 1403–1413.

99 Zhou, Y., Lin, F., Du, Y., Qin, L., Zhao, Z., Xu, J., & Lei, H. (2009). Grey matter abnormalities in IA : A voxel-based morphometry study. *European Journal of Radiology.* Retrieved from http:// sciencedirect.com

100 Liu, J., Gao, X., Osunde, I., Li, X., Zhou, S.K., Zheng, H., & Li, L. (2010). Increased regional homogeneity in Internet Addiction disorder: A resting state functional magnetic resonance imaging study. *Chinese Medical Journal, 123*(4), 1904–1908.

101 Han, D.H., Kim, Y.S., Lee, Y.S., Min, K.J., & Renshaw, P.F. (2010). Changes in cue induced, prefrontal cortex activity with videogame play. *Cyberpsychology, Behavior and Social Networking, 13*(6), 655–661.

102 Han, D.H., Lyoo, I.K., & Renshaw, P.F. (2012). Differential regional gray matter volumes in patients with on-line game addiction and professional gamers. *Journal of Psychiatry Research 46*(4), 507–515.

103 Ruobing, Q., Xianming, F., & Xiapeng, H. (2008). Functional MRI study of Internet game addiction in adolescents. *Chinese Journal of Stereotactic and Functional Neurosurgery, 4*. Retrieved from http://en.cnki.com

104 Dong, G., De Vito, E., Huang, J., & Du, X. (2012). Diffusion tensor imaging reveals thalamus and posterior cingulate cortex abnormalities in Internet gaming addicts. *Journal of Psychiatric Research, 46*, 1212–1216.

105 Note: Studies clearly indicate that "normal" usage of i-tech in "normal" school children decreases their sensitivity to emotional cues, limiting or losing their abilities to read and hence understand the emotions of others. The implications for those with already compromised socio-emotional development, as seen in spectrum disorders, are vast. (See the work of P. Greenwood.)

106 Blinka, L., & Smahel, D. (2011). Addiction to online role playing games. In K.S. Young, & C.N. Nabuco de Abreu (Eds.), *Internet Addiction* (pp. 73–90). Hoboken, NJ: John Wiley & Sons.

107 Zimmerman, F.J. Christakis, D.A., & Meltzoff, A.N. (2007). Television and DVD/video viewing in children younger than 2 years. *Archives of Pediatric and Adolescent Medicine, 161*, 473–479.

108 Gee, J.P. (2003). *What video games have to teach us about literacy and learning*. NY, NY: Palgrave Macmillan.

109 Grizzard, M., Tamborini, R., Lewis, R.J. Wang, L., Prabhu, S. (2014). Being bad in a video game can make us more morally sensitive. *Cyberpsychol Behavior and Social Networking 17*(8):499–504. doi: 10.1089/cyber.2013.0658

110 Kuhl, P.K. (2007). Is speech learning "gated' by the social brain? *Developmental Science, 10 (1)*110–120.

111 Kuhl, P.K., Tsao, F-M., & Liu, H-M. (2003). Foreign-language experience in infancy: Effects of short-term exposure and social interaction on phonetic learning. *Proceedings of the National Academy of Sciences 10* (15), 9096–9101.

112 Sigman, A. (2005). Remotely controlled. London, UK: Random House.

113 Uhlmann, E., & Swanson, J. (2004). Exposure to violent videogames increases automatic aggressiveness. *Journal of Adolescence, 27*, 41–52.

114 Grizzard, M., Tamborini, R., Lewis, R.J. Wang, L., Prabhu, S. (2014). Being bad in a video game can make us more morally sensitive. *Cyberpsychol Behavior and Social Networking 17*(8):499–504. doi: 10.1089/cyber.2013.0658

115 http://isabelagranic.com/interview-benefits-of-playing-video-games/

116 Kuhl, P.K. (2007). Is speech learning "gated' by the social brain? *Developmental Science,* 10 (*1*)110–120.

117 Kuhl, P.K., Tsao, F-M., & Liu, H-M. (2003). Foreign-language experience in infancy: Effects of short-term exposure and social interaction on phonetic learning. *Proceedings of the National Academy of Sciences 10* (15), 9096–9101.

118 Prensky, M. (2001). Digital Natives, Digital Immigrants, Part One. *On the Horizon, 9*(5), 1–6.

119 Bauerlein, M. (Ed) (2011). *The Digital Divide.* London, UK: Penguin

120 Spiral blog: A blog wherein an individual publicly diaries/blogs their descent or demise and finds a readership following (support) based on the negative or the downfall.

121 http://www.niemanlab.org/2011/09/community-planit-turns-civic-engagement-into-a-game-and-the-prize-is-better-discourse/

122 Mueller, P.A. & Oppenheimer, D.M, (2014). The pen is mightier than the keyboard: Advantages of longhand over laptop note taking. *Psychological Science, June 2014; vol. 25,* 6: pp. 1159–1168.

123 O'Callaghan, T. (2014). Digital Technology is transforming the way we read and write: Does it matter. *New Scientist, 224* 2993, pp 41–43.

124 Lubar, J. F., & Shouse, M. N. (1976). EEG and behavioral changes in a hyperactive child concurrent with training of the sensorimotor rhythm (SMR): A preliminary report. *Biofeedback & Self-Regulation, 1*(3), 293–306.

125 Lubar, J. O., & Lubar, J. F. (1984). Electroencephalographic biofeedback of SMR and beta for treatment of attention deficit disorders in a clinical setting. *Biofeedback & Self-Regulation, 9,* 1–23

126 Quenqua, D. (2014). Is e-reading to your toddler story time, or simply screen time? *New York Times*. October 12.

127 Zimmerman, F.J. Christakis, D.A., & Meltzoff, A.N. (2007). Television and DVD/video viewing in children younger than 2 years. *Archives of Pediatric and Adolescent Medicine, 167*, 473–479.

128 See the multiple works of work of Alison Gopnik.

129 Lampit, A., Hallock, H, & Valenzuela, M. (2014).Computerized Cognitive

Training in Cognitively Healthy Older Adults: A Systematic Review and Meta-Analysis of Effect Modifiers Published: November 18, 2014, DOI: 10.1371/journal.pmed.1001756

130 Boot, W.R., Blakely, D.P. and Simons, D.J. (2011) Do Action Video Games Improve Perception and Cognition? *Frontiers in Psychology*, 2011; DOI: 10.3389/fpsyg.2011.00226

131 Neufeld, G., & Maté, G. (2004). *Hold on to your kids*. Toronto, Canada: Random House.

132 Ibid.

133 Ibid.

134 Lamb, S. & Brown, L.M. (2006). *Packaging girlhood.* New York, NY: St. Martin's Press

135 Sigman, A. (2007). Psychologist warns of educational television myth. *Epoch Times,* Feb 21–27, p 14.

136 Sigman, A. (2007). *Remotely controlled*. Canada: Random House.

137 Porges, S. (2011). *The polyvagal theory: Neurophysiological foundations of emotions, attachment, communication, and self-regulation.* New York: W. W. Norton & Company.

138 Ainsworth, M.D., Blehar, M.C., Waters, E., & Wall, S. (1978). *Patterns of attachment*. Hillsdale, NJ: Erlbaum.

139 Cassidy, J., & Shaver, P.R. (Eds.). (1999). *Handbook of attachment*. New York, NY: Guilford Press.

140 Porges, S. (2011). *The polyvagal theory: Neurophysiological foundations of emotions, attachment, communication, and self-regulation.* New York: W. W. Norton & Company.

141 Seigel, D. J. (2001). Toward an interpersonal neurobiology of the developing mind: Attachment relationships, "mindsight," and neural integration. *Infant Mental Health Journal, 22*(1–2), 67–94.

142 Shore, A. (2001). The effects of early relational trauma on right brain development, affect regulation, and infant mental health. *Infant Mental Health Journal, 22*(1), 201–269.

143 Porges, S. (2011). *The polyvagal theory: Neurophysiological foundations of emotions, attachment, communication, and self-regulation.* New York: W. W. Norton & Company.

144 Bellieni, C.V., Cordelli, D.M., Raffaelli, M., Ricci, B., Morgese, G., & Buonocore, G. (2006). Analgesic effect of watching TV during venipuncture. *Archives of Disease in Childhood, 91*, 1015–1017.

145 Christakis, D.A., Zimmerman, F.J., DiGiueppe, D.L., & McCarty, C.A.

(2004). Early television exposure and subsequent attentional problems in children. *Pediatrics, 113*(4), 708–713.

146 Christakis, D., & Zimmerman, F. (2007). Violent television viewing during preschool is associated with antisocial behavior during school age. *Pediatrics, 120*(5), 993–999.

147 Christakis, D.A., Zimmerman, F.J., DiGiueppe, D.L., & McCarty, C.A. (2004). Early television exposure and subsequent attentional problems in children. *Pediatrics, 113*(4), 708–713.

148 Dworak, M., Schierl, T., Bruns, T., & Strüder, H. (2007, November). Impact of singular excessive computer game and television exposure on sleep patterns and memory performance of school-aged Children. *Pediatrics, 120*(5), 978–985.

149 Kuhl and Parish-Morris in Quenqua, D. (2014). Is e-reading to your toddler story time, or simply screen time? *New York Times*. October 12.

150 Landhuis, C.E., Poulton, R ., Welch, D., & Hancox, R.J. (2007).Does Childhood Television Viewing Lead to Attention Problems in Adolescence? Results From a Prospective Longitudinal Study *Pediatrics 120* (3), pp. 532–537.

151 Zimmerman, F.J. Christakis, D.A., & Meltzoff, A.N. (2007). Television and DVD/video viewing in children younger than 2 years. *Archives of Pediatric and Adolescent Medicine, 167*, 473–479.

152 Stern, D.N. (1985). *The interpersonal world of the infant.* New York, NY: Basic Books.

153 Rayner, E., Joyce, A., Rose, J., Twyman, M., & Clulow, C. (2005). *Human development* (4th ed.) New York, NY: Routledge.

154 Bowlby, J. (1982). *Attachment and loss: Vol 1. Attachment* (2nd ed.). NY,NY: Basic Books. (Original work published 1969).

155 Shore, A. (2001). The effects of early relational trauma on right brain development, affect regulation, and infant mental health. *Infant Mental Health Journal, 22*(1), 201–269.

156 Lerner, R.M. (1985). *Concepts and theories of human development* (2nd ed.). NY, NY: Random House.

157 Malacrida, C. (2003). *Cold comfort: Mothers, professionals and Attention Deficit Disorder*. Toronto, Canada: University of Toronto Press.

158 Vehrs in Melillo, R. and Leisman, G. (2004). *Neurobehavioral disorders of childhood*. New York New York: Kluwer Academic/ Plenum Publishers.

159 American Academy of Pediatrics (2013). Children, Adolescents and the Media. APA.

160 Huang, G.C., Unger, J.B., Soto, D., Fujimoto, K., Pentz, M.A., Jordan-Marsh, M., Valente, D., & Huang, T.W. Peer influences: The impact of offline and

online friendship networks on adolescent smoking and alcohol use. *Journal of Adolescent Health, 54* (5) 508–514.

161 See David Suzuki the nature of things. http://www.cbc.ca/natureofthings/

162 An excellent synopsis in Whitebread, D. & Bingham, S. (2013).Too much, too young. *NewScientist, 2943*, 28–29.

163 An excellent synopsis of the relative age effect in the 1980s is presented in a paper by R. H. Barnsley available from http://eric.ed.gov/?id=ED306679

164 Some parents and educators did listen and took action holding younger children back for one scholastic year. As the majority did not, however, most ironically, in the big picture this compounded as opposed to solved the problem. An 8- to 12-month gap, in some instances, grew to an 18-month gap. The very young were thus in an even more compromised learning position. The functional learning gap widened.

165 Gavas, J . & Dazat, O. (2011) *Late Bloomers.* Film.

166 Pellis, S. & Pellis, V. (2010). *The playful brain.* New York, NY: Oneworld Publications

167 Ibid.

168 Neufeld, G., & Maté, G. (2004). *Hold on to your kids*. Toronto, Canada: Random House.

169 Przybylski, A.K. (2014). Electronic gaming and psychosocial adjustment. Doi: 10.1542/peds.2013-4021

170 Simmons, R. (2002). *Odd girl out. The hidden culture of aggression in girls.* Orlando, FL: Harcourt.

171 Fillion, K. (2007). How to fix boys: Let them start school later, and yes let them fight and play with toy guns. Interview with child development expert Leonard Sax, *McLean's, 121*(2),42–45

172 Coloroso, B. (2004). *The bully, the bullied and the bystander*. New York, NY: Harper Collins.

173 Neufeld, G., & Maté, G. (2004). *Hold on to your kids*. Toronto, Canada: Random House.

174 Ibid.

175 Ibid.

176 Rodkin, P.C., Farmer, T.W., Pearl, R., & Van Acker, R. (2000). Heterogeneity of popular boys: antisocial and prosocial configurations. *Developmental Psychology, 36*,(1), 14–24.

177 Simmons, R. (2002). *Odd girl out. The hidden culture of aggression in girls.* Orlando, FL: Harcourt.

178 Cooper, A., Delmonico, D.L., & Burg, R. (2000). Cybersex users, abusers,

and compulsives: New findings and implications. *Sexual Addiction and Compulsivity, 7*, 5–29.

179 Cooper, A., Delmonico, D.L., & Burg, R. (2000). Cybersex users, abusers, and compulsives: New findings and implications. *Sexual Addiction and Compulsivity, 7*, 5–29.

180 Carnes, P., Delmonico, D.L., & Griffin, E. & Moriarity, J.M. (2007). *In the shadows of the net*. Center City, MI: Hazelden.

181 Sigman, A. (2005). *Remotely controlled*. London, UK: Random House.

182 Struthers, W.M. (2009). *Wired for intimacy*. Downers Grove, IL: Intervarsity Press.

183 Shaffer, H.J. (1996). Understanding the means and objects of addiction: Technology, the Internet and gambling. *Journal of Gambling Studies, 12*(4), 461-469.

184 Swingle, M. (2013). *Electroencephalographic (EEG) brainmap patterns in a clinical sample of adults diagnosed with an Internet addiction*. PhD Dissertation. Fielding Graduate University.

185 Carnes, P., Delmonico, D.L., & Griffin, E. & Moriarity, J.M. (2007). *In the shadows of the net*. Center City, MI: Hazelden.

186 Schneider, J.P. (2000). A qualitative study of cybersex participants; Gender differences, recovery issues, and implications for therapists. *Sexual Addiction and Compulsivity: The Journal of Treatment and Prevention, 7*(4), 249–278.

187 Struthers, W.M. (2009). *Wired for intimacy*. Downers Grove, IL: Intervarsity Press.

188 Wolf, N. (2003). The porn myth. *New York Magazine, 20*. Retrieved from http:// nymag.com

189 Cooper, A., Delmonico, D.L., & Burg, R. (2000). Cybersex users, abusers, and compulsives: New findings and implications. *Sexual Addiction and Compulsivity, 7*, 5–29.

190 Carnes, P., Nonemaker, D., & Skilling, N. (1991). Gender differences in normal and sexually addicted populations. *American Journal of Preventative Psychiatry and Neurology, 3*, 16–23.

191 Struthers, W.M. (2009). *Wired for intimacy*. Downers Grove, IL: Intervarsity Press.

192 Wolf, N. (2003). The porn myth. *New York Magazine, 20*. Retrieved from http:// nymag.com

193 Raymond, N.C., Coleman, E., & Miner, M.H. (2003). Psychiatric comorbidity and compulsive/impulsive traits in compulsive sexual behavior. *Comprehensive Psychiatry, 44,* 370–380.

194 Kafka, M. (2000). Psychopharmacological treatments for nonparaphilic compulsive sexual behaviors. *CNS Spectrums, 5*, 49–59.

195 Karim, R. (2009). Cutting edge pharmacology for sex addiction: How do the meds work? A presentation for the Society for the Advancement of Sexual Health, San Diego, CA.

196 Raymond, N.C., Grant, J.E., Kim, S.W., & Coleman, E. (2002). Treating compulsive sexual behavior with naltrexone and serotonin reuptake inhibitors: Two case studies. *International Clinical Psychopharmacology,* 17, 201–205.

197 Linden, D.J. (2011). *The Compass of Pleasure*. New York, NY: Penguin.

198 Doidge, N. (2007). *The Brain That Changes Itself: Stories of Personal Triumph from the Frontiers of Brain Science*. London, UK: Penguin.

199 Small, G. & Vorgan, G. (2008). iBrain: Surviving the technological alteration of the modern mind. New York, NY: Harper Collins.

200 Uhls, Y.T., Michikanyan, M., Garcia, J., Small, G.W., Zgourou, E., & Greenfield. (2014). Five days at outdoor education camp without screens improves preteen skills with nonverbal emotion cues. *Computers in Human Behavior, 39*, 387–392.

201 Chatfield, T. (2015). *Netymology: From Apps to Zombies: A linguistic celebration of the digital age.* London, UK: Quercus Publishing.

202 Turkle, S. (2011). *Alone together: Why we expect more from technology and less from each other.* New York, NY: Basic Books.

203 Rosen, L. (2012). *iDisorder.* New York, NY: Palgrave Macmillan.

204 Dunbar, R. (2014). Friendship: Do animals have friends, too? *NewScientist, 2970*, 34–36.

205 Small, G. & Vorgan, G. (2008). iBrain: Surviving the technological alteration of the modern mind. New York, NY: Harper Collins.

206 Baraniuk, C. (2014). Digital courts rule. *New Scientist, 15* (21), p 22.

207 Oppenheimer, T. (2003). *The flickering mind: The false promise of technology in the classroom and how learning can be saved*. New York, NY: Random House.

208 Young, K.S., & Nabuco de Abreu, C. N. (Eds.). (2011). *Internet addiction.* Hoboken, NJ: John Wiley & Sons.

209 Block, J.J. (2008). Issues for DSM-V: IA. *American Journal of Psychiatry, 165*, 306–307.

210 Shaw, M.Y., & Black, D.W. (2008). Internet addiction: Definition, assessment, epidemiology and clinical management. *CNS Drugs, 22*, 353–365.

211 Cooper, A., Delmonico, D.L., & Burg, R. (2000). Cybersex users, abusers, and compulsives: New findings and implications. *Sexual Addiction and Compulsivity, 7*, 5–29.

212 Donovan, D.M. (1988). Assessment of addictive behaviors: Implications of an emerging biopsychosocial model. In D.M. Donovan & G.A. Marlat (Eds.), *Assessment of addictive behaviors* (pp. 3–50). New York, NY: Guilford Press.

213 American Psychiatric Association (APA). (2000). *Diagnostic and statistical manual of mental* disorders (4th ed., text revision). Arlington, VA: Author.

214 American Society of Addiction Medicine (ASAM). (2011). Public policy statement: Definition of addiction. Retrieved from http://www.asam.org

215 Orzack, M.H. (1999). Computer addiction: Is it real or virtual? *Harvard Mental Health Letter, 15*(7), 8.

216 Block, J.J. (2008). Issues for DSM-V: IA. *American Journal of Psychiatry, 165*, 306–307.

217 Young, K.S., Yue, D.X., & Ying, L. (2011). Prevalence estimates and etiologic models of Internet addiction. In K.S. Young, & C.N. Nabuco de Abreu (Eds.) *Internet addiction* (pp.3–17). Hoboken, NJ: John Wiley & Sons.

218 Greenfield, D.N. (1999). Psychological characteristics of compulsive Internet use: A preliminary analysis. *CyberPsychology and Behavior, 8*(5), 403-412

219 Swingle, M. (2013). *Electroencephalographic (EEG) brainmap patterns in a clinical sample of adults diagnosed with an Internet addiction*. PhD Dissertation. Fielding Graduate University.

220 Griffiths, M. (2000b). IA. Time to be taken seriously. *Addiction Research, 8*(5), 413–418.

221 Cooper, A., Delmonico, D.L., & Burg, R. (2000). Cybersex users, abusers, and compulsives: New findings and implications. *Sexual Addiction and Compulsivity, 7*, 5–29.

222 Suller, J. (2004). The online disinhibition effect. *Cyber Psychology and Behavior, 7*(3), 321–326.

223 Griffiths, M. (2000a). Does Internet and computer addiction exist? Some case study evidence. *CyberPsychology and Behavior, 3*(2), 211–218.

224 Greenfield, D.N. (1999). Psychological characteristics of compulsive Internet use: A preliminary analysis. *CyberPsychology and Behavior, 8*(5), 403–412.

225 Young, K. S. (1998). *Caught in the net: How to recognise the signs of Internet addiction and a winning strategy for recovery.* New York, NY: John Wiley & Sons.

226 Young, K. (2011). Clinical assessment of Internet-addicted clients. In K.S. Young & C. Nabuco de Abreu (Eds.), *Internet addiction* (pp. 19–34). Hoboken, NJ: Wiley.

227 Young, K.S. (1998). IA: The emergence of a new clinical disorder. *CyberPsychology and Behavior, 1*(3), 237–244.

228 Young, K.S., & Nabuco de Abreu, C. N. (Eds.). (2011). *Internet addiction.* Hoboken, NJ: John Wiley & Sons.

229 Ferraro, G., Caci, B., D'Amico, A., & Di Blasi, M. (2007). Internet Addiction disorder: An Italian study. *CyberPsychology and Behavior, 10*(2), 170–175.

230 Khazaal, Y., Billieux, J., Thorens, G., Khan, R., Louati. Y., Scarlatti., E., Theintz, F., Lederrey, J., Van Der Linden, M., & Zullino, D. (2008). French validation of the Internet Addiction Test. *CyberPsychology and Behavior, 11*(6), 703–706.

231 Widyanto, L., & McMurren, M. (2004). The psychometric properties of the Internet Addiction Test. *CyberPsychology and Behavior, 7*(4), 445–453.

232 Cheon, K.A., Ryu, Y.H., Kim, Y.K., Namkoong, K., Kim, C.H., & Lee, J.D. (2003). Dopamine transporter density in the basal ganglia in children assessed with attention deficit hyperactivity. *European Journal of Nuclear Medicine, 30,* 306-311.

233 Ahmad Agil quoted in Knapton, S. (2014). Study links obesity and gadgets: Nighttime use of TVs, ipads and computers affects metabolism. *Vancouver Sun*. Oct. 4.

Dr. Mari Swingle holds an BA in Visual Arts from University of Ottawa, (1987), MA in Language Education from the University of British Columbia (1997), and a MA and PhD in Clinical Psychology from Fielding Graduate University (2013). She is a BCIA Fellow (2010) and a practicing clinician, Certified Neurotherapist (since 2000). Dr. Mari, as she is known in her practice, is the 2015 winner of the Association for Applied Psychophysiology and Biofeedback (AAPB) Federation of Associations in Behavioral and Brain Sciences (FABBS) Foundation Early Career Impact Award for her research on the effects of i-technology on brain function. Dr. Mari presents her research and speaks regularly on the topic of i-media on the neurophysiology of children and adults.